The Healthy Diet Cookbook for Beginners

Quick and Easy Recipes to Lower Blood Pressure and Boost Heart Health

PHYLIS.R.STOVALL

Copyright © by PHYLIS.R.STOVALL 2024.

All rights reserved. Before this document is duplicated or reproduced in any manner, the publisher's consent must be gained. Therefore, the contents within can neither be stored electronically, transferred, nor kept in database. Neither in Part nor full can the document be copied, scanned, faxed, or retained without approval from the publisher or creator.

TABLE OF CONTENTS

INTRODUCTION 9

Understanding the DASH Diet 11

The Basics of the DASH Diet 13

Benefits of the DASH Diet 17

Essential Ingredients 21

Pantry Staples 27

Equipments and Cooking Techniques 33

    Essential Equipment for the DASH Diet Kitchen 33

    Cooking Techniques for the DASH Diet 37

Shopping List 41

Ingredients Substitution Chart 49

Food to Include, Limit or Avoid 51

    Foods to Include 51

    Foods to Limit 53

    Foods to Avoid 54

Healthy Breakfast Recipes 55

    Avocado and Egg Toast 55

    Greek Yogurt Parfait 56

Spinach and Feta Omelette 56

Banana and Almond Butter Smoothie 57

Oatmeal with Chia and Berries 57

Scrambled Eggs with Tomatoes and Onions 58

Chia Seed Pudding 59

Whole Grain Pancakes with Berries 59

Cottage Cheese with Fruit 60

Sweet Potato Hash with Eggs 61

Apple Cinnamon Quinoa 61

Veggie Breakfast Muffins 62

Almond Butter Banana Toast 63

Green Smoothie 63

Overnight Oats with Almonds 64

Light Lunch Recipes 65

Grilled Chicken Salad 65

Quinoa and Veggie Bowl 66

Turkey and Avocado Wrap 66

Chickpea Salad 67

Grilled Salmon with Asparagus 68

Spinach and Feta Stuffed Chicken Breast 68

Veggie Stir-Fry with Tofu 69

Avocado Tuna Salad 70

Hummus and Veggie Pita 70

Shrimp and Veggie Skewers 71

Zucchini Noodles with Pesto 72

Sweet Potato and Black Bean Salad 72

Grilled Veggie Wrap 73

Cauliflower Fried Rice 74

Avocado Chickpea Toast 74

Snacks and Appetizer Recipes 77

Cucumber and Hummus Bites 77

Baked Sweet Potato Chips 77

Avocado Toast with Cherry Tomatoes 78

Carrot and Celery Sticks with Greek Yogurt Dip 79

Roasted Chickpeas 79

Apple Slices with Almond Butter 80

Guacamole with Whole Wheat Crackers 80

Caprese Skewers 81

Cucumber and Feta Salad 82

Zucchini Fries 82

Roasted Veggie Bites 83

Greek Yogurt with Berries 84

Edamame with Sea Salt 84

Mini Veggie Quesadillas 85

Veggie and Cheese Skewers 85

Delicious Dinner Recipes 87

Grilled Chicken with Quinoa and Veggies 87

Baked Salmon with Asparagus 87

Turkey and Sweet Potato Stir-Fry 88

Zucchini Noodles with Marinara Sauce 89

Grilled Shrimp with Brown Rice and Spinach 89

Lentil and Vegetable Stew 90

Spaghetti Squash with Pesto and Cherry Tomatoes 91

Chicken and Vegetable Stir-Fry 92

Baked Cod with Roasted Vegetables 92

Quinoa and Black Bean Salad 93

Grilled Veggie Tacos 94

Turkey Meatballs with Roasted Brussels Sprouts 94

Eggplant Parmesan 95

Beef and Vegetable Skewers 96

Chicken and Avocado Salad 96

Sweet Desserts Recipes 99

Greek Yogurt Parfait with Berries 99

Baked Apple with Cinnamon 99

Banana Oatmeal Cookies 100

Chia Seed Pudding 101

Dark Chocolate Almond Bark 101

Coconut Macaroons 102

Avocado Chocolate Mousse 103

Berry Sorbet 103

Pear with Cinnamon and Walnuts 104

Pumpkin Spice Energy Bites 104

Raspberry Coconut Bars 105

Almond Flour Cookies 106

Frozen Banana Bites 106

Ricotta Cheese with Honey and Almonds 107

Chocolate Dipped Strawberries 107

Healthy Vegetarian Recipes 109

Quinoa Salad with Roasted Vegetables 109

Spinach and Chickpea Stir-Fry 109

Zucchini Noodles with Pesto ... 110

Lentil Soup ... 111

Sweet Potato and Black Bean Tacos ... 111

Grilled Veggie Wrap ... 112

Cauliflower Rice Stir-Fry ... 113

Eggplant Parmesan ... 113

Chickpea Salad ... 114

Vegetable Frittata ... 115

Roasted Brussels Sprouts with Balsamic Vinegar ... 115

Avocado and Tomato Salad ... 116

Sweet Potato and Kale Salad ... 117

Butternut Squash Soup ... 117

Tofu Scramble ... 118

Fruits and Smoothies Recipes ... 119

Mango and Spinach Smoothie ... 119

Berry Blast Smoothie ... 119

Tropical Avocado Smoothie ... 120

Green Apple and Kale Smoothie ... 121

Watermelon Mint Smoothie ... 121

Peach and Banana Smoothie ... 122

Pineapple Coconut Smoothie 122

Strawberry Banana Smoothie 123

Blueberry and Oat Smoothie 124

Mixed Berry Chia Smoothie 124

Kiwi and Pineapple Smoothie 125

Apple Cinnamon Smoothie 125

Papaya Coconut Smoothie 126

Orange and Carrot Smoothie 127

Cucumber Mint Smoothie 127

Exercises and Tips 129

BONUS 133

90 Days Healthy Meal Plan 133

INTRODUCTION

Are you looking for a simple, effective way to improve your health, feel energized, and make better food choices without feeling overwhelmed? If so, you're in the right place. The **Healthy Dash Diet Cookbook for Beginners** is your perfect guide to starting a lifestyle that not only supports heart health but also helps you manage blood pressure, boost energy, and create delicious meals that nourish your body from the inside out.

The DASH (Dietary Approaches to Stop Hypertension) diet isn't just another trendy diet; it's a well-researched eating plan backed by science, designed specifically to help reduce high blood pressure and improve overall wellness. And the best part? It's easy to follow and doesn't require restrictive rules or complicated meal plans. Instead, it focuses on real, whole foods that are rich in nutrients, packed with flavor, and incredibly satisfying.

In this cookbook, we've made the DASH diet approachable and enjoyable for anyone, whether you're new to healthy eating or looking to make a change in your current diet. We understand that starting something new can feel intimidating, but with simple, straightforward recipes and helpful tips, you'll quickly feel confident in your ability to prepare meals that support your health goals. Each recipe is designed with beginners in mind, so there's no need to stress over unfamiliar ingredients or complicated cooking techniques.

Throughout this book, you'll discover the power of fresh fruits, vegetables, lean proteins, whole grains, and healthy fats. These are the building blocks of the DASH diet, and they'll quickly become the foundation of your daily meals. But it's not just about the food you eat—it's about feeling good in your body, taking control of your health, and building lasting habits that fit seamlessly into your lifestyle.

Understanding the DASH Diet

The **DASH Diet**—which stands for **Dietary Approaches to Stop Hypertension**—is not just another trendy eating plan; it's a lifestyle that focuses on improving heart health, lowering blood pressure, and enhancing overall well-being. Developed by nutrition experts and backed by years of research, the DASH diet has been proven to help people manage high blood pressure and reduce the risk of heart disease. But even more than that, it's a simple, sustainable approach to healthy eating that everyone can benefit from, regardless of age or health status.

At its core, the DASH diet emphasizes **whole, nutrient-rich foods** that are naturally low in sodium and high in essential vitamins, minerals, and fiber. It's about making healthier food choices without feeling deprived or resorting to overly complicated meals. The key to success on the DASH diet is focusing on the right balance of foods—fruits, vegetables, whole grains, lean proteins, and low-fat dairy—while cutting back on foods that can contribute to high blood pressure, such as foods high in sodium, saturated fats, and added sugars.

The Key Principles of the DASH Diet

1. **Focus on Nutrient-Dense Foods**: The DASH diet encourages the consumption of foods that are packed with nutrients but low in calories. This includes a wide variety of **fruits** and **vegetables**—aiming for at least 4–5 servings of each per day. Potassium, magnesium, and fiber are abundant in these foods and are necessary for sustaining normal blood pressure levels.

2. **Whole Grains are a Must**: The diet emphasizes **whole grains** like brown rice, quinoa, whole wheat, and oats over refined grains. Whole grains are not only a great source of fiber but also help stabilize blood sugar levels, which can prevent cravings and overeating.

3. **Lean Proteins**: Protein is an important part of the DASH diet, but it's about making healthy choices. Focus on lean meats, such as **poultry** and **fish**, and plant-based sources like **beans**,

lentils, and **tofu**. These provide essential amino acids without the added saturated fats found in some red meats.

4. **Low-Fat Dairy**: Low-fat or fat-free dairy products, such as **milk**, **yogurt**, and **cheese**, are important components of the DASH diet. These foods provide a rich source of calcium and vitamin D, which help support bone health and overall wellness, without the extra saturated fats.

5. **Limit Sodium**: One of the central goals of the DASH diet is to reduce **sodium** intake. The diet encourages staying within the recommended daily limit of 1,500 milligrams of sodium, which is about two-thirds of a teaspoon of salt. This helps lower blood pressure and reduce the risk of heart disease.

6. **Healthy Fats**: Unlike some diets that completely cut out fats, the DASH diet encourages **healthy fats**, like those from **olive oil**, **avocados**, and **nuts**. These fats support heart health and are a better option than saturated fats, which are commonly found in fatty meats and full-fat dairy products.

7. **Limit Sweets and Sugary Drinks**: The DASH diet also encourages limiting foods and drinks that are high in added sugars, like **sodas**, **sweets**, and processed snacks. Instead, you'll focus on naturally sweet options like **fresh fruit**, which can help satisfy your cravings without the negative health impacts.

The Benefits of the DASH Diet

Adopting the DASH diet isn't just about lowering blood pressure—it's about creating a lasting, healthier lifestyle. Studies have shown that the DASH diet can significantly lower blood pressure, improve cholesterol levels, and reduce the risk of heart disease and stroke. It can also help with **weight management**, promote **digestive health**, and support better **blood sugar control**, making it ideal for people with diabetes or those at risk.

The Basics of the DASH Diet

The **DASH Diet** (Dietary Approaches to Stop Hypertension) is based on simple, yet powerful principles designed to help you make healthier food choices that support overall well-being, with a particular focus on reducing high blood pressure. Unlike fad diets that promise quick fixes, the DASH diet offers a sustainable way of eating that promotes heart health, weight management, and disease prevention for life.

At its core, the DASH diet encourages eating **whole, unprocessed foods** while limiting unhealthy options like those high in sodium, saturated fats, and added sugars. It's all about balance—providing your body with essential nutrients from a variety of food groups to ensure you're fueling it with what it needs to thrive.

Here's a breakdown of the core elements of the DASH diet:

1. Focus on Fruits and Vegetables

One of the key principles of the DASH diet is to **fill your plate with fruits and vegetables**. These foods are naturally rich in vitamins, minerals, and fiber, which are essential for good health. They also provide **potassium**, which helps balance the effects of sodium on blood pressure, and **magnesium**, another important mineral for heart health.

- **Recommended servings**: 4-5 servings of fruits and 4-5 servings of vegetables per day.
- **Tips**: Keep your plate colorful! The more vibrant, the better. Fresh, frozen, or canned (without added salt or sugar) options work well.

2. Whole Grains over Refined Grains

The DASH diet encourages the consumption of **whole grains**, which provide a higher level of fiber and nutrients compared to refined grains like white bread and pasta. Fiber is crucial for digestion, keeping blood sugar levels steady, and supporting heart health.

- **Recommended servings**: 6-8 servings of grains per day, with at least half being whole grains.
- **Examples**: Brown rice, quinoa, whole-wheat bread, and oats are excellent choices.

3. Lean Proteins

Protein is a vital part of a healthy diet, but the DASH diet emphasizes **lean protein** sources, which are lower in unhealthy fats. Protein helps build and repair tissue, maintain muscle mass, and keep you feeling full longer.

- **Recommended servings**: 2 or fewer servings of lean meat, poultry, or fish per day, along with plant-based protein sources like beans, lentils, tofu, and nuts.
- **Examples**: Grilled chicken, salmon, eggs, beans, and legumes.

4. Low-Fat or Fat-Free Dairy

Dairy products, especially those that are low in fat or fat-free, are a rich source of **calcium** and **vitamin D**, both of which are important for bone health and managing blood pressure. The DASH diet includes dairy but encourages options that are lower in saturated fats.

- **Recommended servings**: 2-3 servings of low-fat or fat-free dairy products per day.
- **Examples**: Skim milk, fat-free yogurt, and low-fat cheese.

5. Healthy Fats

The DASH diet doesn't eliminate fats; instead, it focuses on choosing **healthy fats** that support heart health. These fats can help reduce cholesterol and inflammation, which are key factors in preventing heart disease.

- **Recommended servings**: 2-3 servings of healthy fats per day.
- **Examples**: Olive oil, avocados, and nuts like almonds, walnuts, and flaxseeds.

6. Limit Sodium and Added Sugars

A critical aspect of the DASH diet is reducing **sodium** intake, as high sodium levels can lead to high blood pressure. The general recommendation is to limit sodium to 1,500–2,300 milligrams per day, or about half a teaspoon of salt. The DASH diet also suggests cutting back on added sugars, which can contribute to weight gain and increase the risk of chronic diseases.

- **Sodium**: Focus on fresh foods and use herbs and spices instead of salt to add flavor.
- **Sugar**: Limit sugary snacks, sodas, and processed foods.

7. Moderation with Sweets and Alcohol

While the DASH diet doesn't ban sweets entirely, it encourages enjoying them in **moderation**. It also recommends limiting alcohol intake, as excessive alcohol can raise blood pressure and contribute to weight gain.

- **Sweets**: Keep to 5 or fewer servings per week.
- **Alcohol**: Limit alcohol to one drink per day for women and two for men.

8. Hydration

Water is essential for good health and maintaining proper bodily functions. The DASH diet encourages drinking plenty of water throughout the day. While water is the healthiest choice, unsweetened beverages like herbal teas can also be included.

The DASH Diet Servings Breakdown

The DASH diet is flexible, but it does offer general guidelines on how many servings of each food group to aim for daily, depending on your calorie needs. Here's a quick overview for a **2,000-calorie** per day plan:

- **Fruits**: 4-5 servings

- **Vegetables**: 4-5 servings
- **Grains**: 6-8 servings
- **Lean protein**: 2 or fewer servings
- **Dairy**: 2-3 servings
- **Four to five servings of nuts, seeds, and legumes each week**
- **Fats and oils**: 2-3 servings
- **Sweets**: 5 or fewer servings per week

Getting Started with the DASH Diet

Starting the DASH diet doesn't require a complete overhaul of your eating habits overnight. Begin by gradually incorporating more fruits, vegetables, whole grains, and lean proteins into your meals. Swap out higher-sodium options for fresher, less processed alternatives. Most importantly, don't stress about perfection—focus on progress.

By understanding and following the basics of the DASH diet, you can reduce your risk of high blood pressure, boost your overall health, and enjoy delicious meals that support your lifestyle. It's a simple, sustainable way of eating that can truly transform the way you feel day after day.

Benefits of the DASH Diet

The **DASH Diet** (Dietary Approaches to Stop Hypertension) is more than just a heart-healthy eating plan—it's a well-rounded approach that provides numerous health benefits, both short-term and long-term. Developed to reduce high blood pressure, the DASH diet has been shown to improve heart health, manage weight, and lower the risk of chronic diseases. Below are some of the key benefits that come with adopting the DASH diet:

1. Lowers Blood Pressure

The DASH diet was specifically designed to **lower high blood pressure**, making it an effective tool for those managing hypertension. By focusing on nutrient-rich, potassium-packed foods, such as fruits and vegetables, and cutting back on sodium, the DASH diet helps balance blood pressure levels. Studies have shown that people following the DASH diet experience significant reductions in both systolic and diastolic blood pressure.

- **How it works**: The diet's emphasis on **potassium**, **magnesium**, and **calcium**—minerals known to help regulate blood pressure—along with its **low sodium** approach, helps to reduce tension in blood vessels and improve circulation.

2. Supports Heart Health

Beyond just lowering blood pressure, the DASH diet is great for overall **heart health**. By cutting out processed foods, refined grains, and excess sodium, while promoting heart-healthy fats, lean proteins, and fiber-rich foods, the DASH diet supports a **healthy cardiovascular system**.

- **Reduced cholesterol levels**: The DASH diet encourages eating foods that are low in unhealthy fats and high in healthy fats, which can reduce LDL (bad) cholesterol levels and raise HDL (good) cholesterol levels.

- **Reduced risk of heart disease and stroke**: Research has found that the DASH diet can significantly lower the risk of **stroke**, **heart disease**, and other cardiovascular conditions.

3. Aids in Weight Loss and Weight Management

The DASH diet can also support healthy **weight loss** and **weight management**. While weight loss isn't the primary focus of the DASH diet, it naturally encourages a reduction in calorie intake by promoting portion control and the consumption of nutrient-dense foods that keep you fuller longer.

- **Balanced meals**: By eating whole grains, fruits, vegetables, lean proteins, and healthy fats, you'll feel satisfied with fewer calories.
- **Healthy habits**: The DASH diet promotes healthy eating habits that can be sustained over time, which is key for maintaining a healthy weight in the long term.

4. Lowers the Chance of Type 2 Diabetes

Diabetes management benefits from the DASH diet as well. It helps regulate **blood sugar levels** by promoting the consumption of fiber-rich foods, lean proteins, and low-glycemic index carbohydrates. This balanced approach helps keep blood sugar levels stable, which is particularly important for individuals with type 2 diabetes or those at risk of developing it.

- **How it helps**: The diet's emphasis on whole grains, legumes, and fiber helps regulate glucose metabolism and reduces insulin resistance.

5. Improves Kidney Function

A diet rich in potassium, calcium, and magnesium, as well as low in sodium, can improve **kidney health**. For people with mild kidney issues or those looking to prevent kidney disease, following the DASH diet can help maintain proper kidney function.

- **How it works**: By avoiding excess sodium, the DASH diet helps reduce the burden on the kidneys, allowing them to function more effectively.

6. Enhances Overall Well-Being

While the DASH diet is primarily known for its heart and blood pressure benefits, it also promotes **overall health**. The diet's high fiber content, along with a rich variety of vitamins and minerals, supports digestive health, boosts energy, and helps improve mood.

- **Digestive health**: The high fiber from fruits, vegetables, and whole grains helps prevent constipation and supports a healthy digestive system.

- **Mental clarity and mood**: A well-balanced diet that supports blood sugar levels and nutrient intake can also have a positive impact on mood and cognitive function, helping you feel more energized and focused.

7. Reduces the Risk of Certain Cancers

While research is ongoing, there is evidence to suggest that the DASH diet may help **reduce the risk of certain cancers**. The diet's emphasis on plant-based foods, which are rich in antioxidants, may help protect cells from damage caused by free radicals, a factor in the development of cancer. Moreover, the diet's focus on limiting red meats, processed foods, and sugars, which are linked to certain types of cancer, can further reduce cancer risk.

- **Plant-based foods**: The abundant fruits, vegetables, and legumes in the DASH diet provide valuable antioxidants, which support cellular health and may lower cancer risk.

8. Promotes Bone Health

By focusing on **low-fat dairy** and other calcium-rich foods, the DASH diet can play a significant role in promoting **bone health** and reducing the risk of osteoporosis. Calcium, along with vitamin D and magnesium, is essential for strong bones, and the DASH diet provides an excellent balance of these nutrients.

- **How it helps**: The DASH diet supports strong bones by providing sufficient calcium and magnesium, which are essential for bone density and preventing bone-related conditions.

9. Improves Skin Health

The DASH diet's emphasis on fruits, vegetables, and healthy fats can also have a positive impact on **skin health**. Foods rich in vitamins, minerals, and antioxidants help nourish the skin, protect it from damage, and promote a youthful appearance.

- **Skin-friendly foods**: The diet's focus on hydrating fruits and vegetables, healthy fats like those found in avocados, and antioxidant-rich foods can help reduce the appearance of wrinkles and improve overall skin health.

Essential Ingredients

1. Fruits

Fruits are a cornerstone of the DASH diet, packed with potassium, antioxidants, vitamins, and fiber. They help lower blood pressure, boost energy, and support overall health.

- **Bananas**: A great source of potassium, which helps balance sodium and regulate blood pressure.

- **Berries**: Blueberries, strawberries, raspberries, and blackberries are full of antioxidants, fiber, and vitamin C.

- **Oranges**: Rich in vitamin C and potassium, which aid in lowering blood pressure.

- **Apples**: High in fiber and antioxidants, apples help manage weight and promote digestive health.

- **Avocados**: A healthy source of fats and potassium, avocados support heart health and provide essential nutrients.

2. Vegetables

Vegetables, especially leafy greens, provide essential vitamins, minerals, and fiber. They are low in calories and packed with nutrients, which contribute to healthy blood pressure and overall wellness.

- **Spinach**: High in potassium, magnesium, and fiber, spinach helps support heart health and healthy blood pressure.

- **Kale**: Rich in vitamin K, calcium, and potassium, kale is a superfood that supports bone and heart health.

- **Sweet Potatoes**: A fiber-rich root vegetable that's high in potassium, helping to manage blood pressure and provide lasting energy.

- **Broccoli**: Packed with fiber, vitamins, and minerals, including potassium and magnesium, which support cardiovascular health.

- **Carrots**: High in fiber and beta-carotene, carrots promote healthy digestion and provide antioxidants.

3. Whole Grains

Whole grains are a key component of the DASH diet, offering fiber, vitamins, and minerals that support heart health and blood sugar control.

- **Brown Rice**: A whole grain that's high in fiber and helps regulate blood sugar levels.

- **Oats**: Oats are rich in soluble fiber, which helps reduce cholesterol and improve heart health.

- **Quinoa**: A high-protein, gluten-free whole grain that contains all nine essential amino acids.

- **Whole Wheat Bread**: A source of fiber that helps manage blood sugar levels and keeps you fuller for longer.

- **Barley**: A fiber-rich grain that supports digestive health and helps lower cholesterol levels.

4. Lean Proteins

The DASH diet emphasizes lean protein sources to help support muscle repair and overall health while keeping fat intake to a minimum.

- **Chicken Breast**: A low-fat protein that provides essential amino acids without excess saturated fat.

- **Turkey**: Another lean source of protein that's versatile for various dishes.

- **Fish**: Salmon, tuna, and other fatty fish are rich in heart-healthy omega-3 fatty acids, which can help lower blood pressure and reduce inflammation.

- **Beans and Legumes**: Kidney beans, black beans, lentils, and chickpeas are great plant-based protein sources full of fiber and essential nutrients.

- **Tofu**: A plant-based protein that's low in fat and can easily absorb the flavors of other ingredients.

5. Low-Fat Dairy or Dairy Alternatives

Dairy provides calcium and vitamin D, which are important for maintaining bone health and managing blood pressure.

- **Skim Milk**: A fat-free source of calcium and vitamin D to help keep bones strong and manage blood pressure.

- **Low-Fat Yogurt**: High in probiotics, calcium, and protein, low-fat yogurt supports digestive health and helps balance blood pressure.

- **Almond Milk**: A dairy-free alternative that's often fortified with calcium and vitamin D.

- **Greek Yogurt**: A thicker, higher-protein yogurt that supports gut health and is rich in calcium.

6. Healthy Fats

Healthy fats are important for heart health and overall well-being, especially when consumed in moderation.

- **Olive Oil**: Rich in monounsaturated fats, which help lower LDL cholesterol and reduce inflammation.

- **Nuts: Pistachios, walnuts, and almonds are rich in protein, fiber, and good fats.** They help reduce bad cholesterol and improve heart health.

- **Chia Seeds**: Packed with omega-3 fatty acids and fiber, chia seeds help support heart health and digestion.

- **Flaxseeds**: An excellent source of omega-3s, fiber, and antioxidants that promote cardiovascular health.

7. Herbs and Spices

Herbs and spices not only enhance the flavor of your meals but also provide valuable nutrients without adding sodium or unhealthy fats.

- **Garlic**: Known for its ability to lower blood pressure and cholesterol levels, garlic also adds depth of flavor.

- **Cilantro**: Rich in antioxidants and vitamin K, cilantro supports detoxification and digestion.

- **Basil**: High in vitamin K and magnesium, basil is great for heart health and reducing inflammation.

- **Turmeric**: Known for its anti-inflammatory properties, turmeric supports joint health and improves circulation.

- **Cinnamon**: Helps stabilize blood sugar levels and adds a sweet flavor without the need for added sugar.

8. Legumes and Beans

These plant-based proteins are a great alternative to meat and provide fiber, protein, and essential minerals like potassium and magnesium.

- **Chickpeas**: Rich in fiber, protein, and iron, chickpeas support digestion and provide long-lasting energy.

- **Black Beans**: Full of fiber, antioxidants, and protein, black beans are great for heart health and managing blood sugar.

- **Lentils**: High in protein and fiber, lentils help regulate blood sugar levels and promote digestive health.

9. Hydration

Water is the most important nutrient your body needs, and staying hydrated supports all of your body's vital functions, including digestion, circulation, and temperature regulation. Staying hydrated also helps with kidney function and overall heart health.

- **Water**: Drinking sufficient water throughout the day is key to staying hydrated and supporting overall health.

- **Herbal Teas**: Unsweetened herbal teas like chamomile, peppermint, and ginger provide hydration while offering additional health benefits.

10. Sweets (in Moderation)

While the DASH diet limits sweets, it allows small amounts of naturally sweet treats, especially when they are made with healthy ingredients.

- **Dark Chocolate**: Rich in antioxidants and lower in sugar, dark chocolate can be a satisfying treat in moderation.

- **Berries**: Naturally sweet, berries can be a great way to satisfy a sweet craving while boosting your nutrient intake.

Pantry Staples

1. Whole Grains

Whole grains are a cornerstone of the DASH Diet. They are packed with fiber, which aids digestion, helps manage cholesterol levels, and keeps you feeling fuller longer.

- **Brown Rice**: A versatile, fiber-rich grain that can be used in a variety of dishes, from stir-fries to casseroles.

- **Quinoa**: A high-protein, gluten-free grain that provides essential amino acids and can be used as a base for salads, soups, or as a side dish.

- **Oats**: Ideal for breakfast, oats are rich in soluble fiber and can be used in oatmeal, smoothies, or as an ingredient in baked goods.

- **Whole Wheat Pasta**: A healthier alternative to regular pasta, providing more fiber and nutrients.

- **Barley**: A hearty grain that's great for soups, stews, and salads. It promotes intestinal health and has a high fiber content.

---

2. Legumes and Beans

Legumes are an excellent plant-based source of protein, fiber, and essential minerals like potassium and magnesium. They're perfect for adding to salads, soups, stews, and casseroles.

- **Canned or Dried Beans**: Kidney beans, black beans, garbanzo beans (chickpeas), and lentils are great pantry options for protein-packed meals. Always opt for low-sodium varieties or rinse canned beans to reduce sodium intake.

- **Split Peas**: Great for making soups, split peas are rich in fiber and protein.

- **Canned Lentils**: Convenient and quick, canned lentils are a great protein source for salads or curries.

---

3. Nuts and Seeds

Nuts and seeds are healthy sources of fats, protein, and fiber, providing the body with essential nutrients. They can be used in smoothies, snacks, salads, or as toppings for dishes.

- **Almonds**: High in heart-healthy fats, almonds are perfect for snacking or adding to oatmeal and salads.
- **Walnuts**: Rich in omega-3 fatty acids, walnuts are great for heart health and can be added to baked goods or sprinkled on salads.
- **Chia Seeds**: Packed with omega-3s and fiber, chia seeds are ideal for adding texture to smoothies, yogurt, or overnight oats.
- **Flaxseeds**: Ground flaxseeds are rich in fiber and omega-3s. They can be sprinkled on cereals, yogurt, or added to baking recipes.
- **Sunflower Seeds**: These seeds are a great snack and provide a good source of magnesium and vitamin E.

---

4. Canned Goods

Canned foods can be a convenient way to stock up on healthy ingredients without sacrificing nutrition. Just make sure to choose options with no added salt or sugar whenever possible.

- **A pantry staple for preparing stews, soups, and sauces is canned tomatoes.** Opt for no-salt-added varieties.

- **Canned Tuna (in water)**: A lean protein option for quick salads, sandwiches, or casseroles. Be sure to choose tuna packed in water to keep the fat content lower.

- **Canned Beans**: As mentioned earlier, canned beans are a pantry staple for easy, protein-packed meals.

- **Canned Corn**: A great addition to salads, soups, and salsas.

- **Canned Artichokes**: Perfect for adding to Mediterranean-inspired dishes, or tossing in salads.

---

5. Spices and Herbs

Herbs and spices are vital for flavoring DASH-friendly meals without adding excess salt. They also provide numerous health benefits, such as anti-inflammatory properties and improved digestion.

- **Garlic Powder**: Adds flavor without the sodium of table salt.

- **Ground Turmeric**: Known for its anti-inflammatory benefits, turmeric can be added to curries, soups, and smoothies.

- **Cumin**: A warm, earthy spice that's perfect for adding depth to soups, stews, and vegetable dishes.

- **Paprika**: Adds a smoky, slightly sweet flavor to meals like roasted vegetables or chicken.

- **Dried Oregano**: A must-have for Mediterranean-inspired dishes and a key ingredient in Italian cuisine.

- **Cinnamon**: Great for adding flavor to baked goods, oatmeal, or smoothies without added sugar.

6. Healthy Oils and Vinegars

Healthy oils provide essential fats and are crucial for cooking and making dressings. Vinegars add a burst of flavor to salads and marinades, without extra calories or sodium.

- **Olive Oil**: Rich in heart-healthy monounsaturated fats, olive oil is ideal for cooking, drizzling on salads, or making homemade dressings.

- **Avocado Oil**: Another heart-healthy oil with a high smoke point, perfect for roasting, grilling, or stir-frying.

- **Apple Cider Vinegar**: Known for its health benefits, apple cider vinegar can be used in salad dressings, marinades, or to add acidity to dishes.

- **Balsamic Vinegar**: A sweet and tangy vinegar that pairs wonderfully with olive oil in dressings and marinades.

---

7. Whole Grain Flours

Whole grain flours provide more fiber and nutrients than refined white flour. They're great for baking, making pancakes, or thickening sauces.

- **Whole Wheat Flour**: Ideal for making whole grain bread, pancakes, muffins, and more.

- **Almond Flour**: A gluten-free option that's perfect for baking low-carb or gluten-free treats.

- **Oat Flour**: Made from ground oats, oat flour can be used for pancakes, muffins, or as a thickener for soups and sauces.

- **Chickpea Flour**: A gluten-free option that's high in protein and fiber, great for savory dishes or baking.

8. Low-Sodium Broths and Stocks

Low-sodium broths and stocks are essential for making soups, stews, and sauces without adding excess salt.

- **Chicken Broth (Low-Sodium)**: A base for soups, casseroles, or sauces, chicken broth is a must-have for DASH-friendly recipes.

- **Vegetable Broth**: Perfect for plant-based dishes, vegetable broth adds flavor without too much sodium.

- **Beef Broth (Low-Sodium)**: Another great option for making hearty stews and sauces with less salt.

9. Sweeteners (in Moderation)

While the DASH diet limits sugar intake, small amounts of natural sweeteners can be used to satisfy your sweet tooth without overloading on added sugars.

- **Honey**: A natural sweetener with antioxidants that can be used in tea, smoothies, or dressings.

- **Pure Maple Syrup**: A plant-based sweetener that pairs well with oatmeal or pancakes.

- **Stevia**: A calorie-free sweetener derived from plants, perfect for sweetening beverages and baked goods.

10. Canned or Frozen Vegetables

Stocking up on frozen or canned vegetables is a convenient way to have nutrient-rich options on hand when fresh produce isn't available.

- **Frozen Peas, Corn, or Mixed Vegetables**: These are quick and easy to add to soups, casseroles, or stir-fries.

- **Frozen Spinach**: An excellent source of iron and vitamins, frozen spinach can be easily added to soups, smoothies, and sauces.

- **Canned Pumpkin**: Great for adding to soups, smoothies, or baking. It's rich in fiber and beta-carotene.

Equipments and Cooking Techniques

Essential Equipment for the DASH Diet Kitchen

Equipping your kitchen with the right tools can make preparing DASH Diet meals both easier and more enjoyable. With these essential kitchen items, you'll have everything you need to create healthy, flavorful meals that align with the principles of the DASH Diet. Here's a list of must-have equipment to have on hand:

1. Non-Stick Cookware

Non-stick pans are a game-changer for healthier cooking, allowing you to use less oil while still getting excellent results. A well-equipped kitchen should include:

- **Non-Stick Frying Pan**: Great for sautéing vegetables, cooking eggs, and pan-frying lean proteins like chicken or fish with minimal oil.

- **Non-Stick Saucepan**: Ideal for simmering soups, stews, and sauces. It makes cleanup easy and reduces the need for added fats.

- **Non-Stick Baking Sheets**: Perfect for roasting vegetables, baking fish, or making low-fat baked goods without sticking.

2. Slow Cooker (Crockpot)

A slow cooker is one of the most useful tools in the kitchen for preparing healthy, low-sodium meals with minimal effort. The slow cooking process allows flavors to develop while keeping the dish low in fat and sodium.

- **Slow Cooker**: Perfect for making stews, soups, beans, and whole grains like quinoa. Simply add your ingredients in the morning, and by dinnertime, you'll have a healthy meal ready to serve.

3. Steamer

Steaming is one of the healthiest cooking methods, as it helps retain the maximum nutrients in vegetables, fish, and even whole grains.

- **Steamer Basket**: If you don't have a dedicated steamer, a simple steamer basket that fits into a saucepan can be used to steam vegetables, fish, or dumplings.

- **Electric Steamer**: For bigger meals, an electric steamer can quickly steam large batches of vegetables or fish while preserving their nutritional value.

4. Blender or Food Processor

A good blender or food processor is essential for making smoothies, soups, sauces, and even dough. These tools help you blend fruits, vegetables, and whole grains into easy-to-digest meals.

- **High-Powered Blender**: Perfect for making smoothies, blending vegetables into sauces, or pureeing soups for a creamy texture.

- **Food Processor**: Ideal for chopping vegetables, grinding nuts or seeds, or preparing homemade dips like hummus.

5. Mandoline Slicer

A mandoline slicer allows for precise slicing of fruits and vegetables, making it easier to prepare salads, stir-fries, and casseroles with uniform slices.

- **Mandoline Slicer**: Excellent for thinly slicing vegetables like zucchini, cucumbers, carrots, and sweet potatoes. It helps save time and ensures even cooking.

6. Grater

A simple kitchen tool that is versatile for shredding vegetables, cheese (in moderation), or zesting fruits for extra flavor.

- **Box Grater or Microplane**: Use for grating carrots, zucchini, and cheese or zesting lemon or orange for added flavor without added sodium.

7. Baking Pans and Loaf Pans

For anyone baking DASH-friendly treats or making heart-healthy dishes like casseroles or loaves, having a variety of baking pans is essential.

- **Glass or Ceramic Baking Dish**: Use these for casseroles, roasted vegetables, or even low-fat baked pasta dishes.

- **Loaf Pan**: Perfect for making whole grain breads or healthy baked goods, like banana bread or zucchini bread.

8. Instant Pot

An Instant Pot is a multi-functional pressure cooker that can save time and effort in preparing healthy meals. It's perfect for cooking whole grains, beans, lean meats, and vegetables quickly.

- **Instant Pot**: Its one-pot cooking capability can help you create hearty soups, stews, and even yogurt, making it a versatile addition to your DASH Diet kitchen.

9. Sharp Knives

Having sharp, high-quality knives in your kitchen will make chopping vegetables, cutting meats, and preparing meals much easier and more efficient.

- **Chef's Knife**: A good-quality chef's knife is the workhorse of your kitchen. It's essential for slicing, dicing, and chopping all your ingredients.
- **Paring Knife**: A smaller, more delicate knife, great for peeling and trimming fruits and vegetables.

10. Measuring Cups and Spoons

The DASH Diet emphasizes portion control, so having an accurate set of measuring cups and spoons ensures that you're not overeating or adding too much of any ingredient.

- **Measuring Cups**: Use for liquids and dry ingredients like flour, oats, and rice. They help ensure you stick to proper portions.
- **Measuring Spoons**: Essential for adding spices, salt substitutes, and small amounts of liquids like oil or vinegar.

11. Cutting Board

A large, sturdy cutting board provides a clean surface for chopping and slicing. It also prevents cross-contamination between raw meats and vegetables.

- **Wooden or Plastic Cutting Board**: Opt for multiple boards—one for meats and one for vegetables, to avoid any contamination.

12. Tongs and Wooden Spoons

Tongs and wooden spoons are essential tools for stir-frying, sautéing, or flipping ingredients during cooking.

- **Tongs**: Great for flipping meats, stirring vegetables, and serving.
- **Wooden Spoons**: Ideal for stirring soups, sauces, and stews without scratching non-stick pans.

Cooking Techniques for the DASH Diet

Now that you have the right tools, it's time to focus on the healthy cooking techniques that align with the **DASH Diet** principles. These techniques emphasize reducing sodium, fats, and calories while maximizing flavor and nutrients.

1. Roasting

Roasting is a great way to bring out the natural sweetness of vegetables while keeping them healthy and low in fat. Simply toss vegetables with a small amount of olive oil and your favorite herbs and spices, then roast in the oven at a high temperature.

- **Tips**: Avoid using excessive oil, and try roasting in batches to save time. Roasted veggies like Brussels sprouts, sweet potatoes, or carrots can be added to salads, bowls, or served as a side.

2. Grilling

Grilling is a fantastic way to cook lean proteins like chicken, fish, and vegetables without needing much added fat. It imparts a smoky flavor that enhances natural tastes.

- **Tips**: Always marinate proteins with herbs, citrus, and olive oil to add flavor without salt. Avoid sugary marinades that can increase calorie intake.

---

3. Sautéing

Sautéing is perfect for cooking vegetables, lean proteins, and whole grains in a small amount of oil or broth. This method retains nutrients while enhancing flavors.

- **Tips**: Use heart-healthy oils like olive oil or avocado oil. Always start with a hot pan, so food cooks quickly and evenly.

---

4. Steaming

Steaming is one of the healthiest ways to cook vegetables, fish, and even whole grains. It preserves nutrients while maintaining a fresh, natural taste.

- **Tips**: Steam your vegetables lightly to keep them crisp and colorful. Use a dash of lemon or vinegar to elevate the flavor without sodium.

---

5. Slow Cooking

Slow cooking is ideal for soups, stews, and chili. It allows flavors to meld together over several hours while keeping meals low in fat and sodium.

- **Tips**: Choose lean cuts of meat and add plenty of vegetables and legumes for a filling and nutrient-packed meal.

6. Baking

Baking isn't just for sweet treats—it's perfect for making low-fat casseroles, healthy breads, and even roasted fish or chicken.

- **Tips**: Opt for whole grains in your baking, and use healthier substitutes for sugar and fats (like applesauce or yogurt) to keep things DASH-friendly.

Shopping List

Fruits and Vegetables

Fresh fruits and vegetables are at the heart of the DASH Diet. Aim to include a wide variety of colorful produce in your meals.

- **Fruits**:
  - Apples
  - Bananas
  - Berries (strawberries, blueberries, raspberries)
  - Oranges
  - Pears
  - Grapes
  - Pineapple
  - Avocados
  - Mangoes
  - Kiwi
- **Vegetables**:
  - Leafy greens (spinach, kale, arugula, lettuce)
  - Carrots
  - Bell peppers (red, yellow, green)
  - Tomatoes
  - Cucumbers
  - Zucchini

- Broccoli
- Cauliflower
- Brussels sprouts
- Sweet potatoes
- Green beans
- Asparagus
- Mushrooms

Whole Grains

Whole grains are an excellent source of fiber, vitamins, and minerals that support heart health.

- **Grains**:
  - Brown rice
  - Quinoa
  - Oats (rolled oats or steel-cut oats)
  - Whole wheat pasta
  - Whole wheat bread
  - Whole grain tortillas
  - Bulgur
  - Barley
  - Farro

Proteins

Lean proteins are a key part of the DASH Diet, providing essential nutrients without added saturated fats.

- **Meat and Poultry**:
  - Skinless chicken breast or thighs
  - Lean cuts of beef (round, sirloin)
  - Lean pork pieces, such as loin chops and tenderloin
  - Turkey (ground, breast)
- **Fish and Seafood**:
  - Salmon
  - Tuna (fresh or canned in water)
  - Trout
  - Shrimp
  - Cod
  - Sardines
- **Plant-Based Proteins**:
  - Lentils
  - Chickpeas
  - Black beans
  - Kidney beans
  - Tofu
  - Tempeh
  - Edamame

Dairy

Low-fat and fat-free dairy options provide calcium and vitamin D to support bone health.

- **Dairy Products**:

- Skim or 1% milk
- Low-fat or fat-free yogurt
- Low-fat or fat-free cheese (cheddar, mozzarella, ricotta)
- Cottage cheese (low-fat)

Healthy Fats

Incorporate healthy fats into your diet, including those from plant-based sources like nuts, seeds, and oils.

- **Healthy Oils**:
    - Olive oil
    - Avocado oil
    - Canola oil
    - Coconut oil (in moderation)
- **Nuts and Seeds**:
    - Almonds
    - Walnuts
    - Cashews
    - Chia seeds
    - Flaxseeds
    - Sunflower seeds
    - Pumpkin seeds
- **Nut Butters**:
    - Natural peanut butter
    - Almond butter

Herbs and Spices

Flavor your meals with fresh herbs and dried spices to enhance taste without adding sodium.

- **Fresh Herbs**:
    - Basil
    - Cilantro
    - Parsley
    - Dill
    - Mint
    - Rosemary
    - Thyme
- **Dried Spices**:
    - Garlic powder
    - Onion powder
    - Black pepper
    - Ground cinnamon
    - Paprika
    - Cumin
    - Chili powder
    - Turmeric
    - Oregano
    - Ginger
- **Salt Substitutes**:
    - Mrs. Dash (salt-free seasoning)

- Lemon zest
- Vinegar (balsamic, apple cider)

Legumes

Legumes are rich in fiber and protein and can be used in soups, salads, or as a meat alternative.

- **Legumes**:
    - Canned or dried beans (black, kidney, garbanzo, pinto)
    - Lentils (green, brown, red)
    - Split peas
    - Edamame (fresh or frozen)

Beverages

Choose beverages that complement a healthy, low-sodium lifestyle.

- **Beverages**:
    - Herbal teas (green, chamomile, peppermint)
    - Coffee (limit sugar and cream)
    - Sparkling water
    - 100% fruit juices (in moderation, no added sugar)
    - Coconut water

Miscellaneous

Other essentials for cooking and meal preparation.

- **Whole Wheat Flour**
- **Low-Sodium Vegetable or Chicken Broth**

- **Low-Sodium Canned Tomatoes**
- **Vinegar (balsamic, apple cider)**
- **Unsweetened Applesauce**
- **Whole Wheat Crackers**
- **Low-Sodium Canned Beans**
- **Almond milk without sugar (or other plant-based milks)**

Ingredients Substitution Chart

Original Ingredient	Substitute	Reason for Substitution
Butter	Olive oil, avocado, or coconut oil	Lower in saturated fat and provides healthy fats.
Heavy cream	Unsweetened almond milk or low-fat milk	Lower in fat and calories, while still creamy.
Whole milk	Skim milk or unsweetened plant-based milk	Lower in saturated fat and calories.
Full-fat cheese	Reduced-fat cheese or nutritional yeast	Lower in fat and calories while maintaining flavor.
Sour cream	Greek yogurt (plain, non-fat)	Higher in protein and lower in fat.
Mayonnaise	Greek yogurt (plain, non-fat) or hummus	Provides creaminess with lower fat and more protein.
Sugar	Honey, stevia, or maple syrup (in moderation)	Natural sweeteners with lower glycemic index and fewer calories.
White flour	Whole wheat flour or almond flour	Higher in fiber and nutrients, better for blood sugar control.
Regular pasta	Whole wheat pasta or zucchini noodles	Higher in fiber, lower glycemic index, and more nutrients.
White rice	Brown rice or quinoa	Higher in fiber and nutrients, helping with blood sugar management.
Bacon	Turkey bacon or lean ham	Lower in saturated fat and sodium.

Original Ingredient	Substitute	Reason for Substitution
Ground beef (80% lean)	Ground turkey or lean ground chicken	Lower in saturated fat, calories, and cholesterol.
Regular sausage	Turkey sausage or plant-based sausage	Lower in saturated fat, calories, and sodium.
Sweetened yogurt	Unsweetened Greek yogurt + fruit	Lower in added sugars and offers more protein.
Fried foods	Grilled, baked, or roasted alternatives	Lower in unhealthy fats and calories.
Canned beans in syrup	Low-sodium canned beans or dried beans	Lower in sodium and preservatives, higher in fiber and nutrients.
Salt	Herbs and spices (garlic, onion, rosemary, thyme, turmeric)	Reduces sodium while adding flavor and health benefits.
Canned tomato sauce	Fresh tomatoes blended or low-sodium tomato sauce	Reduces sodium while maintaining flavor.
Regular crackers	Whole grain or gluten-free crackers	Higher in fiber, lower in refined carbohydrates.
Regular chips	Baked tortilla chips or veggie chips	Lower in fat and calories, higher in nutrients.
Frozen vegetables with added sauce	Fresh or frozen vegetables with no added sauce	Eliminates unnecessary sodium and preservatives.
Regular salad dressing	Olive oil and vinegar or low-fat dressing	Lower in unhealthy fats and calories.
Regular peanut butter	Natural peanut butter (unsweetened)	Lower in added sugars and unhealthy fats.

Original Ingredient	Substitute	Reason for Substitution
Frozen yogurt	Frozen banana slices or sorbet	Lower in fat and calories, made with natural sweetness.

Food to Include, Limit or Avoid

Foods to Include

These foods can help lower blood pressure and enhance heart health because they are high in vital minerals like potassium, magnesium, calcium, fiber, and antioxidants.

1. Fruits

- Fresh fruits are high in vitamins, fiber, and antioxidants, which are key to supporting cardiovascular health.
  - Apples, bananas, oranges, strawberries, blueberries, grapes, and melon.
  - Avocados (rich in healthy fats and potassium).

2. Vegetables

- Fruits and vegetables are high in fiber, vitamins, and minerals and low in calories.
  - Leafy greens include Swiss chard, collard greens, arugula, spinach, and kale.
  - Cruciferous vegetables: broccoli, cauliflower, Brussels sprouts.
  - Root vegetables: carrots, sweet potatoes, and beets.
  - Allium vegetables: onions, garlic, leeks, and shallots.

3. Whole Grains

- Whole grains are an excellent source of fiber and nutrients, helping to manage weight and promote heart health.
  - Brown rice, quinoa, barley, whole wheat bread, whole grain pasta, oats, and farro.

4. Lean Protein

- Foods high in protein are necessary for both muscle repair and a balanced metabolism.
    - Skinless poultry (chicken and turkey), lean cuts of beef (sirloin, round), and pork (tenderloin).
    - Omega-3 fatty acids fatty acid-rich fish include salmon, tuna, trout, and sardines.
    - Plant-based proteins: lentils, chickpeas, black beans, tofu, tempeh, and edamame.

5. Low-Fat Dairy

- Low-fat dairy provides calcium and vitamin D for strong bones and teeth, as well as protein for muscle maintenance.
    - Skim or 1% milk, low-fat yogurt, low-fat cheese (cheddar, mozzarella), and low-fat cottage cheese.

6. Nuts, Seeds, and Legumes

- Plant-based protein, fiber, and good fats are abundant in nuts, seeds, and legumes.
    - Almonds, walnuts, pistachios, chia seeds, flaxseeds, sunflower seeds, and pumpkin seeds.
    - Beans and legumes like kidney beans, pinto beans, black beans, lentils, and split peas.

7. Healthy Fats

- Nutritious fats lower cholesterol and lessen inflammation.
    - Olive oil, avocado oil, and canola oil for cooking.
    - Avocados (source of healthy monounsaturated fats).

8. Herbs and Spices

- Fresh and dried herbs and spices can add flavor without extra salt.
    - Fresh herbs: parsley, cilantro, basil, thyme, rosemary, oregano, and mint.
    - Dried spices: turmeric, cinnamon, paprika, black pepper, garlic powder, cumin, and chili powder.

9. Beverages

- Hydration is essential for overall health, and low-sodium drinks are encouraged.
    - Water, herbal teas, and unsweetened iced tea.
    - Freshly squeezed juice (in moderation), preferably with no added sugar.
    - Plant-based milks, such as almond milk, that are low in fat or unsweetened.

Foods to Limit

Limiting certain foods ensures you're not consuming excessive sodium, sugar, or unhealthy fats, all of which can contribute to high blood pressure and poor heart health.

1. Sodium

- Sodium increases blood pressure, so it's important to limit high-sodium foods.
    - Avoid processed and packaged foods that are high in salt, such as canned soups, frozen dinners, and salty snacks.
    - Limit the use of salt when cooking; instead, opt for salt-free seasoning blends or herbs.

2. Added Sugars

- Excess sugar intake can contribute to weight gain and an increased risk of heart disease.
    - Limit sugary beverages like soda, fruit juices with added sugar, and energy drinks.
    - Cut back on baked goods and snacks high in sugar, such as cookies, cakes, and candies.
    - Be cautious with flavored yogurts and breakfast cereals, as they often contain added sugars.

3. Red and Processed Meats

- Saturated fats, which can elevate cholesterol and harm heart health, are abundant in these meats.
    - Limit your intake of fatty lamb, pork, and beef cuts.

- Steer clear of processed meats that are high in sodium and bad fats, such as hot dogs, bacon, sausages, and deli meats.

4. Full-Fat Dairy

- Saturated fats, which are abundant in full-fat dairy products, can raise cholesterol levels.
  - Limit full-fat cheese, butter, and whole milk.

5. Fried Foods and Fast Food

- Fried foods frequently include large amounts of calories and harmful trans fats, which raise the risk of heart disease and cause weight gain.
  - Steer clear of deep-fried items like battered fish, fried chicken, and French fries.
  - Limit fast food, which is often high in sodium, unhealthy fats, and empty calories.

Foods to Avoid

Some foods are best avoided altogether on the DASH Diet due to their high content of unhealthy fats, sodium, and sugars.

1. Processed Snacks and Sweets

- Usually, these foods are heavy in sugar, harmful fats, and empty calories.
  - Avoid chips, pretzels, candy bars, cakes, pies, and other packaged snacks that are high in sodium, sugar, and fat.

2. Sugary Beverages

- Sugary drinks are one of the major contributors to weight gain, diabetes, and high blood pressure.
  - Avoid sodas, sugary fruit drinks, and sweetened coffee drinks.

3. Highly Refined Grains

- Refined grains have been stripped of fiber and nutrients and can lead to blood sugar spikes.
  - Avoid white bread, white rice, and regular pasta, as they are made with refined flour.

4. High-Sodium Convenience Foods

- Many convenience foods contain high levels of sodium, which can raise blood pressure.
  - Avoid microwave meals, canned soups, packaged ramen, and pre-seasoned frozen meals.

Healthy Breakfast Recipes

Avocado and Egg Toast

Ingredients:

- 1 slice whole-grain bread
- 1/2 ripe avocado
- 1 large egg
- Salt and pepper to taste
- 1 tsp olive oil

Serving Size: 1 serving
Nutritional Value: 250 calories, 12g protein, 19g fat, 22g carbs, 6g fiber

Prep Time: 5 minutes
Cook Time: 5 minutes

Instructions:

1. Toast the bread.
2. Mash avocado and spread on the toast.
3. Heat olive oil in a pan, fry the egg to your liking.
4. Place the egg on the toast, season with salt and pepper.

Greek Yogurt Parfait

Ingredients:

- 1/2 cup plain Greek yogurt (low-fat)
- 1/4 cup mixed berries (blueberries, strawberries, raspberries)
- 1 tbsp chia seeds
- 1 tsp honey

Serving Size: 1 serving
Nutritional Value: 180 calories, 12g protein, 7g fat, 20g carbs, 6g fiber

Prep Time: 5 minutes
Cook Time: 0 minutes

Instructions:

1. Layer yogurt, berries, chia seeds, and honey in a cup or bowl.
2. Serve immediately.

Spinach and Feta Omelette

Ingredients:

- 2 large eggs
- 1/4 cup spinach, chopped
- 1 tbsp feta cheese, crumbled
- Salt and pepper to taste

Serving Size: 1 serving
Nutritional Value: 210 calories, 16g protein, 14g fat, 2g carbs

Prep Time: 3 minutes
Cook Time: 5 minutes

Instructions:

1. Whisk eggs, salt, and pepper.
2. Heat a non-stick pan and add spinach. Cook for 1-2 minutes.
3. Pour eggs over spinach, cook until set.
4. Sprinkle feta and fold. Serve hot.

Banana and Almond Butter Smoothie

Ingredients:

- 1 medium banana
- 1 tbsp almond butter
- 1/2 cup unsweetened almond milk
- 1/2 tsp cinnamon

Serving Size: 1 serving
Nutritional Value: 210 calories, 5g protein, 14g fat, 23g carbs, 4g fiber

Prep Time: 5 minutes
Cook Time: 0 minutes

Instructions:

1. Blend all ingredients until smooth.
2. Pour into a glass and enjoy.

Oatmeal with Chia and Berries

Ingredients:

- 1/2 cup rolled oats
- 1 cup water or almond milk
- 1 tbsp chia seeds

- 1/4 cup mixed berries
- 1 tsp honey (optional)

Serving Size: 1 serving
Nutritional Value: 220 calories, 6g protein, 7g fat, 31g carbs, 9g fiber

Prep Time: 5 minutes
Cook Time: 5 minutes

Instructions:

1. Cook oats with water or almond milk according to package instructions.
2. Stir in chia seeds and honey.
3. Top with berries and serve.

Scrambled Eggs with Tomatoes and Onions

Ingredients:

- 2 large eggs
- 1/4 cup chopped tomatoes
- 1/4 cup onions, chopped
- Salt and pepper to taste

Serving Size: 1 serving
Nutritional Value: 220 calories, 14g protein, 18g fat, 3g carbs

Prep Time: 5 minutes
Cook Time: 5 minutes

Instructions:

1. Sauté onions and tomatoes in a pan until soft.
2. Whisk eggs, add salt and pepper.
3. Scramble the eggs in the pan until they are done. Serve hot.

Chia Seed Pudding

Ingredients:

- 2 tbsp chia seeds
- 1/2 cup almond milk (unsweetened)
- 1 tsp vanilla extract
- 1 tbsp honey

Serving Size: 1 serving
Nutritional Value: 180 calories, 6g protein, 9g fat, 15g carbs, 10g fiber

Prep Time: 5 minutes
Cook Time: 0 minutes (let sit overnight)

Instructions:

1. Combine honey, almond milk, vanilla, and chia seeds.
2. Refrigerate overnight.
3. Stir and serve with fresh fruit in the morning.

Whole Grain Pancakes with Berries

Ingredients:

- 1/2 cup whole-wheat flour
- 1/2 tsp baking powder
- 1/4 tsp cinnamon
- 1 egg
- 1/2 cup almond milk
- 1/4 cup mixed berries

Serving Size: 2 pancakes
Nutritional Value: 220 calories, 6g protein, 8g fat, 30g carbs, 5g fiber

Prep Time: 5 minutes
Cook Time: 5 minutes

Instructions:

1. Mix flour, baking powder, cinnamon, egg, and almond milk to form a batter.
2. Cook pancakes on a hot griddle until golden, flipping once.
3. Top with fresh berries.

Cottage Cheese with Fruit

Ingredients:

- 1/2 cup low-fat cottage cheese
- 1/2 cup mixed fruit (pineapple, peach, or berries)

Serving Size: 1 serving
Nutritional Value: 180 calories, 12g protein, 5g fat, 18g carbs, 3g fiber

Prep Time: 2 minutes
Cook Time: 0 minutes

Instructions:

1. Combine cottage cheese and fruit.
2. Serve immediately.

Sweet Potato Hash with Eggs

Ingredients:

- 1 medium sweet potato, diced
- 1/4 cup onion, diced
- 1 tsp olive oil
- 1 large egg

Serving Size: 1 serving
Nutritional Value: 250 calories, 7g protein, 12g fat, 30g carbs, 5g fiber

Prep Time: 5 minutes
Cook Time: 15 minutes

Instructions:

1. Sauté sweet potato and onion in olive oil until tender (10-12 minutes).
2. Fry an egg in the same pan and place on top of the hash.
3. Serve hot.

Apple Cinnamon Quinoa

Ingredients:

- 1/2 cup cooked quinoa
- 1/2 apple, diced
- 1/2 tsp cinnamon
- 1 tsp honey

Serving Size: 1 serving
Nutritional Value: 220 calories, 5g protein, 6g fat, 37g carbs, 6g fiber

Prep Time: 5 minutes
Cook Time: 5 minutes

Instructions:

1. Heat cooked quinoa with apple and cinnamon.
2. Drizzle with honey and serve.

Veggie Breakfast Muffins

Ingredients:

- 2 large eggs
- 1/4 cup spinach, chopped
- 1/4 cup bell pepper, chopped
- 1 tbsp feta cheese
- Salt and pepper to taste

Serving Size: 1 muffin
Nutritional Value: 180 calories, 12g protein, 12g fat, 4g carbs

Prep Time: 10 minutes
Cook Time: 15 minutes

Instructions:

1. Preheat oven to 350°F (175°C).
2. Whisk eggs, spinach, bell pepper, and feta.
3. Pour into muffin tin and bake for 15 minutes.

Almond Butter Banana Toast

Ingredients:

- 1 slice whole-grain bread
- 1 tbsp almond butter
- 1/2 banana, sliced
- Cinnamon for sprinkling

Serving Size: 1 serving
Nutritional Value: 250 calories, 8g protein, 14g fat, 28g carbs, 5g fiber

Prep Time: 5 minutes
Cook Time: 0 minutes

Instructions:

1. Toast the bread and spread almond butter.
2. Top with banana slices and sprinkle with cinnamon.

Green Smoothie

Ingredients:

- 1/2 cup spinach
- 1/2 banana
- 1/2 cup unsweetened almond milk
- 1 tbsp chia seeds
- 1/4 cup ice cubes

Serving Size: 1 serving
Nutritional Value: 180 calories, 4g protein, 9g fat, 20g carbs, 8g fiber

Prep Time: 5 minutes
Cook Time: 0 minutes

Instructions:

1. Blend all ingredients until smooth.
2. Pour into a glass and serve.

Overnight Oats with Almonds

Ingredients:

- 1/2 cup rolled oats
- 1/2 cup unsweetened almond milk
- 1 tbsp almond butter
- 1 tbsp sliced almonds
- 1 tsp honey

Serving Size: 1 serving
Nutritional Value: 230 calories, 7g protein, 14g fat, 25g carbs, 5g fiber

Prep Time: 5 minutes
Cook Time: 0 minutes (let sit overnight)

Instructions:

1. Mix oats, almond milk, almond butter, and honey.
2. Refrigerate overnight.
3. Top with sliced almonds before serving.

Light Lunch Recipes

Grilled Chicken Salad

Ingredients:

- Four ounces of grilled and sliced chicken breast
- 2 cups mixed greens (spinach, arugula, romaine)
- 1/4 cup cherry tomatoes, halved
- 1 tbsp olive oil
- 1 tsp balsamic vinegar
- Salt and pepper to taste

Serving Size: 1 serving
Nutritional Value: 290 calories, 28g protein, 16g fat, 6g carbs, 3g fiber

Prep Time: 5 minutes
Cook Time: 10 minutes

Instructions:

1. Grill chicken breast, then slice it.
2. Toss greens and tomatoes with olive oil and balsamic vinegar.
3. Top with chicken, season with salt and pepper.

Quinoa and Veggie Bowl

Ingredients:

- 1/2 cup cooked quinoa
- 1/4 cup cucumber, diced
- 1/4 cup bell pepper, diced
- 1 tbsp olive oil
- 1 tbsp lemon juice
- Salt and pepper to taste

Serving Size: 1 serving
Nutritional Value: 220 calories, 6g protein, 10g fat, 28g carbs, 5g fiber

Prep Time: 5 minutes
Cook Time: 10 minutes (for quinoa)

Instructions:

1. Cook quinoa and let it cool.
2. Mix with cucumber, bell pepper, olive oil, and lemon juice.
3. Season with salt and pepper.

Turkey and Avocado Wrap

Ingredients:

- 4 oz lean turkey breast
- 1 whole wheat wrap
- 1/4 avocado, sliced
- 1/4 cup lettuce, shredded
- 1 tbsp mustard

Serving Size: 1 serving
Nutritional Value: 280 calories, 26g protein, 14g fat, 20g carbs, 7g fiber

Prep Time: 5 minutes
Cook Time: 0 minutes

Instructions:

1. Place turkey on the wrap.
2. Add avocado, lettuce, and mustard.
3. Roll up and serve.

Chickpea Salad

Ingredients:

- 1/2 cup canned chickpeas, drained and rinsed
- 1/4 cup cucumber, diced
- 1/4 cup tomato, diced
- 1 tbsp olive oil
- 1 tbsp lemon juice
- Salt and pepper to taste

Serving Size: 1 serving
Nutritional Value: 220 calories, 9g protein, 9g fat, 28g carbs, 7g fiber

Prep Time: 5 minutes
Cook Time: 0 minutes

Instructions:

1. In a bowl, combine the tomato, cucumber, and chickpeas.
2. Sprinkle some lemon juice and olive oil over it.
3. Season with salt and pepper.

Grilled Salmon with Asparagus

Ingredients:

- 4 oz salmon fillet
- 1/2 bunch asparagus, trimmed
- 1 tbsp olive oil
- Salt and pepper to taste

Serving Size: 1 serving
Nutritional Value: 330 calories, 30g protein, 22g fat, 5g carbs, 3g fiber

Prep Time: 5 minutes
Cook Time: 12 minutes

Instructions:

1. Preheat grill to medium-high heat.
2. Brush salmon and asparagus with olive oil, season with salt and pepper.
3. Grill for 6-7 minutes per side, until salmon is cooked through.

Spinach and Feta Stuffed Chicken Breast

Ingredients:

- 1 boneless, skinless chicken breast
- 1/4 cup spinach, cooked and squeezed dry
- 2 tbsp feta cheese
- 1 tsp olive oil
- Salt and pepper to taste

Serving Size: 1 serving
Nutritional Value: 250 calories, 32g protein, 14g fat, 3g carbs, 1g fiber

Prep Time: 10 minutes
Cook Time: 20 minutes

Instructions:

1. Preheat oven to 375°F (190°C).
2. Slice chicken breast to create a pocket.
3. Stuff with spinach and feta, season with salt and pepper.
4. Bake for 20 minutes.

Veggie Stir-Fry with Tofu

Ingredients:

- 4 oz firm tofu, cubed
- 1/2 cup broccoli florets
- 1/4 cup bell pepper, sliced
- 1 tbsp low-sodium soy sauce
- 1 tbsp olive oil
- 1 tsp ginger, grated

Serving Size: 1 serving
Nutritional Value: 220 calories, 15g protein, 16g fat, 12g carbs, 5g fiber

Prep Time: 5 minutes
Cook Time: 10 minutes

Instructions:

1. Heat olive oil in a pan and sauté tofu until golden.
2. Add broccoli, bell pepper, and ginger, cook for 5 minutes.
3. Stir in soy sauce, cook for another 2 minutes.

Avocado Tuna Salad

Ingredients:

- 1/2 can tuna, drained
- 1/4 avocado, mashed
- 1 tbsp Greek yogurt
- 1 tbsp lemon juice
- Salt and pepper to taste

Serving Size: 1 serving
Nutritional Value: 220 calories, 21g protein, 14g fat, 2g carbs, 5g fiber

Prep Time: 5 minutes
Cook Time: 0 minutes

Instructions:

1. Mix tuna, avocado, Greek yogurt, and lemon juice in a bowl.
2. Season with salt and pepper.

Hummus and Veggie Pita

Ingredients:

- 1 whole wheat pita pocket
- 3 tbsp hummus
- 1/4 cup cucumber, sliced
- 1/4 cup tomato, sliced
- 1/4 cup lettuce

Serving Size: 1 serving
Nutritional Value: 280 calories, 9g protein, 12g fat, 34g carbs, 8g fiber

Prep Time: 5 minutes
Cook Time: 0 minutes

Instructions:

1. Cut pita in half and spread hummus inside.
2. Stuff with cucumber, tomato, and lettuce.
3. Serve immediately.

Shrimp and Veggie Skewers

Ingredients:

- 4 oz shrimp, peeled and deveined
- 1/2 bell pepper, cut into chunks
- 1/4 onion, cut into chunks
- 1 tbsp olive oil
- 1 tsp lemon juice
- Salt and pepper to taste

Serving Size: 1 serving
Nutritional Value: 210 calories, 23g protein, 10g fat, 8g carbs, 3g fiber

Prep Time: 10 minutes
Cook Time: 5 minutes

Instructions:

1. Preheat grill to medium-high heat.
2. Thread shrimp, bell pepper, and onion onto skewers.
3. Brush with olive oil and lemon juice, grill for 2-3 minutes per side.

Zucchini Noodles with Pesto

Ingredients:

- 2 medium zucchinis, spiralized
- 1/4 cup pesto sauce
- 1 tbsp pine nuts (optional)
- 1 tbsp parmesan cheese

Serving Size: 1 serving
Nutritional Value: 220 calories, 7g protein, 18g fat, 8g carbs, 3g fiber

Prep Time: 5 minutes
Cook Time: 5 minutes

Instructions:

1. Sauté zucchini noodles in a pan for 2-3 minutes until tender.
2. Toss with pesto sauce, top with pine nuts and parmesan.

Sweet Potato and Black Bean Salad

Ingredients:

- 1 small sweet potato, roasted and diced
- 1/2 cup black beans, rinsed
- 1 tbsp olive oil
- 1 tbsp lime juice
- Salt and pepper to taste

Serving Size: 1 serving
Nutritional Value: 250 calories, 9g protein, 12g fat, 30g carbs, 8g fiber

Prep Time: 10 minutes
Cook Time: 20 minutes (for roasting sweet potato)

Instructions:

1. Roast sweet potato at 400°F (200°C) for 20 minutes.
2. Combine with black beans, olive oil, lime juice, salt, and pepper.

Grilled Veggie Wrap

Ingredients:

- 1 whole wheat wrap
- 1/4 cup zucchini, grilled
- 1/4 cup eggplant, grilled
- 1 tbsp hummus
- 1/4 cup spinach

Serving Size: 1 serving
Nutritional Value: 230 calories, 7g protein, 10g fat, 32g carbs, 8g fiber

Prep Time: 10 minutes
Cook Time: 10 minutes

Instructions:

1. Grill zucchini and eggplant until tender.
2. Spread hummus on the wrap, then add veggies and spinach.
3. Roll up and serve.

Cauliflower Fried Rice

Ingredients:

- 1 cup cauliflower rice
- 1/4 cup peas and carrots, diced
- 1 egg, scrambled
- 1 tbsp low-sodium soy sauce
- 1 tsp sesame oil

Serving Size: 1 serving
Nutritional Value: 180 calories, 10g protein, 9g fat, 18g carbs, 4g fiber

Prep Time: 5 minutes
Cook Time: 8 minutes

Instructions:

1. Sauté peas and carrots in sesame oil.
2. Add cauliflower rice and soy sauce, cook for 5 minutes.
3. Push rice to the side, scramble the egg in the same pan.
4. Stir everything together and serve.

Avocado Chickpea Toast

Ingredients:

- 1 slice whole-grain bread
- 1/4 avocado, mashed
- 1/4 cup canned chickpeas, mashed
- 1 tsp lemon juice
- Salt and pepper to taste

Serving Size: 1 serving
Nutritional Value: 280 calories, 9g protein, 15g fat, 30g carbs, 9g fiber

Prep Time: 5 minutes
Cook Time: 2 minutes (for toasting bread)

Instructions:

1. Toast the bread.

2. Mash avocado and chickpeas, mix with lemon juice, salt, and pepper.

3. Spread on toast and serve.

Snacks and Appetizer Recipes

Cucumber and Hummus Bites

Ingredients:

- 1 cucumber, sliced
- 3 tbsp hummus

Serving Size: 1 serving (8 slices)
Nutritional Value: 100 calories, 3g protein, 6g fat, 10g carbs, 3g fiber

Prep Time: 5 minutes
Cook Time: 0 minutes

Instructions:

1. Slice cucumber into rounds.
2. Top each slice with a small dollop of hummus.

Baked Sweet Potato Chips

Ingredients:

- 1 medium sweet potato, thinly sliced
- 1 tbsp olive oil
- Salt to taste

Serving Size: 1 serving
Nutritional Value: 150 calories, 2g protein, 7g fat, 23g carbs, 3g fiber

Prep Time: 10 minutes
Cook Time: 20 minutes

Instructions:

1. Preheat oven to 400°F (200°C).
2. Toss sweet potato slices with olive oil and salt.
3. Bake for 20 minutes, flipping halfway.

Avocado Toast with Cherry Tomatoes

Ingredients:

- 1 slice whole-grain bread, toasted
- 1/4 avocado, mashed
- 1/4 cup cherry tomatoes, halved
- Salt and pepper to taste

Serving Size: 1 serving
Nutritional Value: 230 calories, 5g protein, 14g fat, 25g carbs, 7g fiber

Prep Time: 5 minutes
Cook Time: 2 minutes (for toasting)

Instructions:

1. Toast the bread.
2. Mash avocado and spread on toast.
3. Top with tomatoes, salt, and pepper.

Carrot and Celery Sticks with Greek Yogurt Dip

Ingredients:

- 1 carrot, cut into sticks
- 1 celery stalk, cut into sticks
- 3 tbsp Greek yogurt
- 1 tsp lemon juice
- Salt and pepper to taste

Serving Size: 1 serving
Nutritional Value: 120 calories, 6g protein, 5g fat, 15g carbs, 4g fiber

Prep Time: 5 minutes
Cook Time: 0 minutes

Instructions:

1. Mix Greek yogurt with lemon juice, salt, and pepper.
2. Serve with carrot and celery sticks for dipping.

Roasted Chickpeas

Ingredients:

- 1 can chickpeas, drained and rinsed
- 1 tbsp olive oil
- 1 tsp paprika
- Salt to taste

Serving Size: 1 serving
Nutritional Value: 150 calories, 8g protein, 5g fat, 22g carbs, 6g fiber

Prep Time: 10 minutes
Cook Time: 25 minutes

Instructions:

1. Preheat oven to 400°F (200°C).
2. Toss chickpeas with olive oil, paprika, and salt.
3. Roast for 25 minutes, shaking halfway through.

Apple Slices with Almond Butter

Ingredients:

- 1 apple, sliced
- 2 tbsp almond butter

Serving Size: 1 serving
Nutritional Value: 220 calories, 4g protein, 18g fat, 22g carbs, 4g fiber

Prep Time: 5 minutes
Cook Time: 0 minutes

Instructions:

1. Slice apple and serve with almond butter for dipping.

Guacamole with Whole Wheat Crackers

Ingredients:

- 1/2 avocado, mashed
- 1 tbsp lime juice
- 1/4 cup diced tomato
- 1/4 cup diced onion
- 6 whole wheat crackers

Serving Size: 1 serving
Nutritional Value: 220 calories, 4g protein, 15g fat, 20g carbs, 7g fiber

Prep Time: 5 minutes
Cook Time: 0 minutes

Instructions:

1. Mix mashed avocado, lime juice, tomato, and onion.
2. Serve with whole wheat crackers.

Caprese Skewers

Ingredients:

- 8 cherry tomatoes
- 8 small mozzarella balls
- 1 tbsp balsamic vinegar
- 1 tsp olive oil

Serving Size: 1 serving (8 skewers)
Nutritional Value: 160 calories, 9g protein, 13g fat, 6g carbs, 2g fiber

Prep Time: 5 minutes
Cook Time: 0 minutes

Instructions:

1. Skewer tomatoes and mozzarella balls.
2. Pour some balsamic vinegar and olive oil over it.

Cucumber and Feta Salad

Ingredients:

- 1 cucumber, diced
- 1/4 cup feta cheese, crumbled
- 1 tbsp olive oil
- 1 tsp lemon juice

Serving Size: 1 serving
Nutritional Value: 140 calories, 6g protein, 12g fat, 7g carbs, 2g fiber

Prep Time: 5 minutes
Cook Time: 0 minutes

Instructions:

1. Mix cucumber, feta, olive oil, and lemon juice.
2. Serve chilled.

Zucchini Fries

Ingredients:

- 1 zucchini, cut into strips
- 1 egg, beaten
- 1/4 cup whole wheat breadcrumbs
- 1 tbsp olive oil
- Salt and pepper to taste

Serving Size: 1 serving
Nutritional Value: 150 calories, 4g protein, 8g fat, 18g carbs, 3g fiber

Prep Time: 10 minutes
Cook Time: 20 minutes

Instructions:

1. Preheat oven to 400°F (200°C).
2. Dip zucchini strips in egg, coat with breadcrumbs, and season with salt and pepper.
3. Bake for 20 minutes.

Roasted Veggie Bites

Ingredients:

- 1/2 cup bell pepper, diced
- 1/2 cup zucchini, diced
- 1 tbsp olive oil
- Salt and pepper to taste

Serving Size: 1 serving
Nutritional Value: 120 calories, 2g protein, 8g fat, 14g carbs, 5g fiber

Prep Time: 5 minutes
Cook Time: 20 minutes

Instructions:

1. Preheat oven to 400°F (200°C).
2. Toss vegetables in olive oil, season with salt and pepper.
3. Roast for 20 minutes.

Greek Yogurt with Berries

Ingredients:

- 1/2 cup Greek yogurt
- 1/4 cup mixed berries (blueberries, raspberries, strawberries)
- 1 tsp honey (optional)

Serving Size: 1 serving
Nutritional Value: 160 calories, 12g protein, 6g fat, 18g carbs, 3g fiber

Prep Time: 5 minutes
Cook Time: 0 minutes

Instructions:

1. Combine Greek yogurt and berries.
2. Drizzle with honey if desired.

Edamame with Sea Salt

Ingredients:

- 1/2 cup edamame, steamed
- 1/2 tsp sea salt

Serving Size: 1 serving
Nutritional Value: 120 calories, 11g protein, 4g fat, 10g carbs, 4g fiber

Prep Time: 5 minutes
Cook Time: 5 minutes

Instructions:

1. Steam edamame for 5 minutes.
2. Sprinkle with sea salt and serve.

Mini Veggie Quesadillas

Ingredients:

- 1 small whole wheat tortilla
- 1/4 cup of mozzarella or cheddar cheese, shredded
- 1/4 cup bell pepper, diced
- 1/4 cup spinach, chopped

Serving Size: 1 serving
Nutritional Value: 200 calories, 8g protein, 10g fat, 22g carbs, 5g fiber

Prep Time: 5 minutes
Cook Time: 5 minutes

Instructions:

1. Heat tortilla in a pan.
2. Add cheese, bell pepper, and spinach to one half of the tortilla.
3. Fold and cook until cheese melts, about 2-3 minutes per side.

Veggie and Cheese Skewers

Ingredients:

- 1/2 cup cherry tomatoes
- 1/4 cup cucumber, sliced
- 1/4 cup mozzarella balls
- 1 tbsp olive oil

Serving Size: 1 serving (6 skewers)
Nutritional Value: 180 calories, 9g protein, 12g fat, 6g carbs, 3g fiber

Prep Time: 5 minutes
Cook Time: 0 minutes

Instructions:

1. Skewer tomatoes, cucumber, and mozzarella balls.
2. Drizzle with olive oil and serve.

Delicious Dinner Recipes

Grilled Chicken with Quinoa and Veggies

Ingredients:

- 1 chicken breast, grilled
- 1/2 cup quinoa, cooked
- 1/2 cup steamed broccoli
- 1 tbsp olive oil
- Salt and pepper to taste

Serving Size: 1 serving
Nutritional Value: 350 calories, 30g protein, 12g fat, 28g carbs, 6g fiber

Prep Time: 10 minutes
Cook Time: 20 minutes

Instructions:

1. Grill chicken breast until fully cooked.
2. Cook quinoa as per package instructions.
3. Steam broccoli.
4. Serve chicken with quinoa and broccoli, drizzle with olive oil.

Baked Salmon with Asparagus

Ingredients:

- 1 salmon fillet
- 1 cup asparagus, trimmed

- 1 tbsp olive oil
- Lemon juice, to taste
- Salt and pepper to taste

Serving Size: 1 serving
Nutritional Value: 320 calories, 26g protein, 20g fat, 10g carbs, 5g fiber

Prep Time: 5 minutes
Cook Time: 20 minutes

Instructions:

1. Preheat oven to 400°F (200°C).
2. Drizzle salmon and asparagus with olive oil, salt, and pepper.
3. Bake for 20 minutes, squeezing lemon juice over salmon.

Turkey and Sweet Potato Stir-Fry

Ingredients:

- 1/2 lb ground turkey
- 1 medium sweet potato, diced
- 1/2 cup bell peppers, diced
- 1 tbsp olive oil
- 1 tbsp low-sodium soy sauce

Serving Size: 1 serving
Nutritional Value: 350 calories, 25g protein, 15g fat, 30g carbs, 6g fiber

Prep Time: 10 minutes
Cook Time: 20 minutes

Instructions:

1. Heat olive oil in a pan, cook turkey until browned.

2. Add diced sweet potato and bell peppers, cook for 10 minutes.
3. Stir in soy sauce and cook for another 5 minutes.

Zucchini Noodles with Marinara Sauce

Ingredients:

- 1 zucchini, spiralized
- 1/2 cup marinara sauce (low-sodium)
- 1 tbsp olive oil
- 1 tbsp fresh basil, chopped
- Salt and pepper to taste

Serving Size: 1 serving
Nutritional Value: 180 calories, 5g protein, 9g fat, 20g carbs, 4g fiber

Prep Time: 5 minutes
Cook Time: 10 minutes

Instructions:

1. Heat olive oil in a pan, sauté zucchini noodles for 5 minutes.
2. Add marinara sauce and cook for another 5 minutes.
3. Top with fresh basil, salt, and pepper.

Grilled Shrimp with Brown Rice and Spinach

Ingredients:

- 6 oz shrimp, peeled and deveined
- 1/2 cup brown rice, cooked
- 1 cup spinach, sautéed

- 1 tbsp olive oil
- Lemon juice, to taste

Serving Size: 1 serving
Nutritional Value: 300 calories, 26g protein, 8g fat, 30g carbs, 6g fiber

Prep Time: 10 minutes
Cook Time: 15 minutes

Instructions:

1. Grill shrimp for 5 minutes until cooked through.
2. Cook brown rice as per package instructions.
3. Sauté spinach in olive oil.
4. Serve shrimp with rice and spinach, drizzle with lemon juice.

Lentil and Vegetable Stew

Ingredients:

- 1/2 cup lentils, dried
- 1 carrot, diced
- 1 celery stalk, diced
- 1/2 onion, diced
- 1 tbsp olive oil
- 4 cups vegetable broth (low-sodium)

Serving Size: 1 serving
Nutritional Value: 280 calories, 15g protein, 7g fat, 45g carbs, 14g fiber

Prep Time: 10 minutes
Cook Time: 30 minutes

Instructions:

1. Heat olive oil in a pot, sauté onion, carrot, and celery for 5 minutes.
2. Add lentils, vegetable broth, and bring to a boil.
3. Simmer for 30 minutes until lentils are tender.

Spaghetti Squash with Pesto and Cherry Tomatoes

Ingredients:

- 1 spaghetti squash
- 1/4 cup pesto sauce (low-fat)
- 1/2 cup cherry tomatoes, halved
- 1 tbsp olive oil

Serving Size: 1 serving
Nutritional Value: 220 calories, 6g protein, 14g fat, 22g carbs, 6g fiber

Prep Time: 10 minutes
Cook Time: 30 minutes

Instructions:

1. Preheat oven to 400°F (200°C). Roast spaghetti squash for 30 minutes.
2. Shred the squash into noodles.
3. Toss squash with pesto, cherry tomatoes, and olive oil.

Chicken and Vegetable Stir-Fry

Ingredients:

- 1 chicken breast, sliced
- 1/2 cup broccoli florets
- 1/2 cup bell peppers, sliced
- 1 tbsp olive oil
- 1 tbsp low-sodium soy sauce

Serving Size: 1 serving
Nutritional Value: 280 calories, 30g protein, 12g fat, 14g carbs, 5g fiber

Prep Time: 10 minutes
Cook Time: 15 minutes

Instructions:

1. Heat olive oil in a pan, cook chicken until browned.
2. Add vegetables and soy sauce, cook for another 5 minutes.

Baked Cod with Roasted Vegetables

Ingredients:

- 1 cod fillet
- 1/2 cup zucchini, sliced
- 1/2 cup bell peppers, diced
- 1 tbsp olive oil
- Lemon juice, to taste

Serving Size: 1 serving
Nutritional Value: 250 calories, 28g protein, 12g fat, 12g carbs, 4g fiber

Prep Time: 5 minutes
Cook Time: 20 minutes

Instructions:

1. Preheat oven to 375°F (190°C). Bake cod for 20 minutes.

2. Toss vegetables with olive oil, roast alongside cod.

3. Drizzle cod with lemon juice before serving.

Quinoa and Black Bean Salad

Ingredients:

- 1/2 cup cooked quinoa
- 1/4 cup black beans, rinsed
- 1/4 cup corn, fresh or frozen
- 1 tbsp olive oil
- 1 tbsp lime juice

Serving Size: 1 serving
Nutritional Value: 270 calories, 10g protein, 9g fat, 35g carbs, 7g fiber

Prep Time: 5 minutes
Cook Time: 0 minutes

Instructions:

1. Mix cooked quinoa, black beans, and corn in a bowl.

2. Drizzle with olive oil and lime juice, toss to combine.

Grilled Veggie Tacos

Ingredients:

- 2 corn tortillas
- 1/2 cup zucchini, sliced
- 1/4 cup bell peppers, sliced
- 1 tbsp olive oil
- 1 tbsp salsa

Serving Size: 1 serving
Nutritional Value: 230 calories, 6g protein, 10g fat, 30g carbs, 6g fiber

Prep Time: 10 minutes
Cook Time: 10 minutes

Instructions:

1. Grill zucchini and bell peppers in olive oil for 5 minutes.
2. Warm tortillas and fill with grilled veggies.
3. Top with salsa and serve.

Turkey Meatballs with Roasted Brussels Sprouts

Ingredients:

- 1/2 lb ground turkey
- 1/2 cup breadcrumbs (whole wheat)
- 1 egg
- 1 cup Brussels sprouts, halved
- 1 tbsp olive oil

Serving Size: 1 serving
Nutritional Value: 300 calories, 28g protein, 14g fat, 20g carbs, 6g fiber

Prep Time: 10 minutes
Cook Time: 20 minutes

Instructions:

1. Preheat oven to 375°F (190°C). Mix turkey, breadcrumbs, and egg, form meatballs.

2. Roast Brussels sprouts with olive oil for 20 minutes.

3. Bake meatballs for 20 minutes.

Eggplant Parmesan

Ingredients:

- 1 eggplant, sliced
- 1/4 cup breadcrumbs (whole wheat)
- 1/4 cup marinara sauce
- 1/4 cup mozzarella cheese, shredded

Serving Size: 1 serving
Nutritional Value: 250 calories, 12g protein, 12g fat, 28g carbs, 7g fiber

Prep Time: 10 minutes
Cook Time: 25 minutes

Instructions:

1. Preheat oven to 375°F (190°C). Bread eggplant slices and bake for 20 minutes.

2. Top with marinara sauce and cheese, bake for another 5 minutes.

Beef and Vegetable Skewers

Ingredients:

- 4 oz lean beef, cubed
- 1/4 cup bell peppers, cubed
- 1/4 cup onions, cubed
- 1 tbsp olive oil
- Salt and pepper to taste

Serving Size: 1 serving
Nutritional Value: 300 calories, 30g protein, 12g fat, 20g carbs, 5g fiber

Prep Time: 10 minutes
Cook Time: 15 minutes

Instructions:

1. Skewer beef and vegetables, drizzle with olive oil.
2. Grill for 15 minutes, turning occasionally.

Chicken and Avocado Salad

Ingredients:

- 1 chicken breast, grilled and sliced
- 1/2 avocado, sliced
- 2 cups mixed greens
- 1 tbsp olive oil
- 1 tbsp lemon juice

Serving Size: 1 serving
Nutritional Value: 320 calories, 28g protein, 18g fat, 12g carbs, 8g fiber

Prep Time: 5 minutes
Cook Time: 10 minutes

Instructions:

1. Grill chicken and slice.

2. Toss mixed greens, avocado, olive oil, and lemon juice.

3. Top with grilled chicken.

Sweet Desserts Recipes

Greek Yogurt Parfait with Berries

Ingredients:

- 1/2 cup plain Greek yogurt
- 1/4 cup berry mixture (raspberries, blueberries, and strawberries)
- 1 tbsp honey
- 1 tbsp chia seeds

Serving Size: 1 serving
Nutritional Value: 180 calories, 10g protein, 5g fat, 25g carbs, 6g fiber

Prep Time: 5 minutes
Cook Time: 0 minutes

Instructions:

1. Layer Greek yogurt with mixed berries in a bowl.
2. Drizzle with honey and sprinkle chia seeds on top.

Baked Apple with Cinnamon

Ingredients:

- 1 medium apple, cored
- 1 tsp cinnamon
- 1 tsp honey
- 1 tbsp chopped walnuts

Serving Size: 1 serving
Nutritional Value: 200 calories, 2g protein, 6g fat, 35g carbs, 6g fiber

Prep Time: 5 minutes
Cook Time: 20 minutes

Instructions:

1. Preheat oven to 350°F (175°C).

2. Core apple and place in a baking dish.

3. Sprinkle with cinnamon, drizzle with honey, and top with walnuts.

4. Bake for 20 minutes until tender.

Banana Oatmeal Cookies

Ingredients:

- 1 ripe banana, mashed
- 1/2 cup oats
- 1/4 tsp vanilla extract
- 1 tbsp dark chocolate chips (optional)

Serving Size: 1 serving (2 cookies)
Nutritional Value: 150 calories, 3g protein, 4g fat, 28g carbs, 4g fiber

Prep Time: 5 minutes
Cook Time: 10 minutes

Instructions:

1. Preheat oven to 350°F (175°C).

2. Mix mashed banana, oats, vanilla, and chocolate chips in a bowl.

3. Form into 6 small cookies and bake for 10 minutes.

Chia Seed Pudding

Ingredients:

- 1/4 cup chia seeds
- 1 cup unsweetened almond milk
- 1 tsp vanilla extract
- 1 tbsp maple syrup

Serving Size: 1 serving
Nutritional Value: 200 calories, 5g protein, 8g fat, 22g carbs, 10g fiber

Prep Time: 5 minutes
Cook Time: 0 minutes (overnight)

Instructions:

1. Combine chia seeds, almond milk, vanilla, and maple syrup in a bowl.
2. Stir well and refrigerate overnight.
3. Stir before serving and enjoy!

Dark Chocolate Almond Bark

Ingredients:

- Two ounces of dark chocolate (70% or more cocoa)
- 1/4 cup almonds, chopped
- 1/4 tsp sea salt

Serving Size: 1 serving (2-3 pieces)
Nutritional Value: 180 calories, 4g protein, 14g fat, 14g carbs, 4g fiber

Prep Time: 5 minutes
Cook Time: 10 minutes

Instructions:

1. Melt dark chocolate in a microwave-safe bowl, stirring every 20 seconds.
2. Stir in almonds and spread onto parchment paper.
3. Sprinkle with sea salt and refrigerate for 10 minutes.

Coconut Macaroons

Ingredients:

- 1 1/2 cups unsweetened shredded coconut
- 2 egg whites
- 1/4 cup honey
- 1 tsp vanilla extract

Serving Size: 1 serving (2 macaroons)
Nutritional Value: 150 calories, 2g protein, 9g fat, 18g carbs, 3g fiber

Prep Time: 5 minutes
Cook Time: 15 minutes

Instructions:

1. Preheat oven to 350°F (175°C).
2. Beat egg whites until stiff peaks form.
3. Fold in coconut, honey, and vanilla.
4. Spoon mixture onto a baking sheet and bake for 15 minutes.

Avocado Chocolate Mousse

Ingredients:

- 1 ripe avocado
- 2 tbsp cocoa powder (unsweetened)
- 1 tbsp maple syrup
- 1/2 tsp vanilla extract

Serving Size: 1 serving
Nutritional Value: 220 calories, 3g protein, 18g fat, 22g carbs, 8g fiber

Prep Time: 5 minutes
Cook Time: 0 minutes

Instructions:

1. Blend avocado, cocoa powder, maple syrup, and vanilla in a blender until smooth.
2. Chill for 30 minutes before serving.

Berry Sorbet

Ingredients:

- One cup of berry mixture (raspberries, blueberries, and strawberries)
- 1 tbsp honey
- 1/4 cup water

Serving Size: 1 serving
Nutritional Value: 100 calories, 1g protein, 0g fat, 25g carbs, 5g fiber

Prep Time: 5 minutes
Cook Time: 0 minutes (freezing time)

Instructions:

1. Blend berries, honey, and water until smooth.

2. Pour mixture into a shallow dish and freeze for 2 hours.
3. Scrape with a fork every 30 minutes to create a sorbet texture.

Pear with Cinnamon and Walnuts

Ingredients:

- 1 pear, sliced
- 1 tsp cinnamon
- 1 tbsp chopped walnuts
- 1 tsp honey

Serving Size: 1 serving
Nutritional Value: 160 calories, 2g protein, 8g fat, 22g carbs, 5g fiber

Prep Time: 5 minutes
Cook Time: 5 minutes

Instructions:

1. Slice pear and sprinkle with cinnamon.
2. Toast walnuts in a dry pan for 3 minutes.
3. Drizzle pear with honey and top with walnuts.

Pumpkin Spice Energy Bites

Ingredients:

- 1/2 cup oats
- 1/4 cup canned pumpkin
- 1 tbsp chia seeds
- 1/4 tsp pumpkin pie spice

- 1 tbsp honey

Serving Size: 1 serving (2 bites)
Nutritional Value: 150 calories, 4g protein, 5g fat, 22g carbs, 4g fiber

Prep Time: 10 minutes
Cook Time: 0 minutes (chilling time)

Instructions:

1. Mix all ingredients in a bowl.
2. Roll into small balls and refrigerate for 30 minutes.

Raspberry Coconut Bars

Ingredients:

- 1/2 cup unsweetened shredded coconut
- 1/2 cup raspberries, mashed
- 1/4 cup oats
- 1 tbsp honey

Serving Size: 1 serving (1 bar)
Nutritional Value: 180 calories, 4g protein, 10g fat, 24g carbs, 5g fiber

Prep Time: 10 minutes
Cook Time: 15 minutes

Instructions:

1. Preheat oven to 350°F (175°C).
2. Mix coconut, raspberries, oats, and honey.
3. Spread mixture into a baking dish and bake for 15 minutes.

Almond Flour Cookies

Ingredients:

- 1 cup almond flour
- 2 tbsp honey
- 1 egg
- 1/4 tsp vanilla extract

Serving Size: 1 serving (2 cookies)
Nutritional Value: 200 calories, 6g protein, 14g fat, 18g carbs, 3g fiber

Prep Time: 5 minutes
Cook Time: 12 minutes

Instructions:

1. Preheat oven to 350°F (175°C).
2. Mix almond flour, honey, egg, and vanilla.
3. Scoop into 6 cookies and bake for 12 minutes.

Frozen Banana Bites

Ingredients:

- 1 banana, sliced
- 1/4 cup dark chocolate chips
- 1 tbsp almond butter

Serving Size: 1 serving (4-5 bites)
Nutritional Value: 150 calories, 3g protein, 10g fat, 20g carbs, 3g fiber

Prep Time: 5 minutes
Cook Time: 0 minutes (freezing time)

Instructions:

1. Slice banana into rounds.
2. Melt dark chocolate and almond butter together.
3. Dip banana slices into chocolate mixture and freeze for 1 hour.

Ricotta Cheese with Honey and Almonds
Ingredients:

- 1/4 cup ricotta cheese
- 1 tsp honey
- 1 tbsp chopped almonds

Serving Size: 1 serving
Nutritional Value: 180 calories, 8g protein, 14g fat, 12g carbs, 3g fiber

Prep Time: 5 minutes
Cook Time: 0 minutes

Instructions:

1. Spoon ricotta into a bowl.
2. Drizzle with honey and top with almonds.

Chocolate Dipped Strawberries
Ingredients:

- 6 strawberries
- 2 oz dark chocolate (70% cocoa)

Serving Size: 1 serving (3 strawberries)
Nutritional Value: 150 calories, 2g protein, 10g fat, 15g carbs, 4g fiber

Prep Time: 5 minutes
Cook Time: 5 minutes

Instructions:

1. Melt dark chocolate in a microwave-safe bowl.
2. Dip strawberries in chocolate and let cool for 10 minutes.

Healthy Vegetarian Recipes

Quinoa Salad with Roasted Vegetables

Ingredients:

- 1 cup cooked quinoa
- One cup of roasted veggies, such as carrots, bell peppers, and zucchini
- 1 tbsp olive oil
- 1 tbsp lemon juice
- 1/4 tsp black pepper

Serving Size: 1 serving
Nutritional Value: 220 calories, 7g protein, 9g fat, 30g carbs, 6g fiber

Prep Time: 10 minutes
Cook Time: 20 minutes (for roasting vegetables)

Instructions:

1. Roast vegetables at 400°F (200°C) for 20 minutes.
2. Toss quinoa with roasted vegetables, olive oil, lemon juice, and pepper.

Spinach and Chickpea Stir-Fry

Ingredients:

- 2 cups spinach, fresh
- 1/2 cup chickpeas, cooked
- 1 tbsp olive oil
- 1 garlic clove, minced

- 1 tbsp lemon juice

Serving Size: 1 serving
Nutritional Value: 150 calories, 7g protein, 7g fat, 18g carbs, 6g fiber

Prep Time: 5 minutes
Cook Time: 5 minutes

Instructions:

1. Heat olive oil in a pan, sauté garlic for 1 minute.
2. Add chickpeas and spinach, cook until spinach wilts.
3. Drizzle with lemon juice before serving.

Zucchini Noodles with Pesto

Ingredients:

- 2 zucchinis, spiralized
- 1/4 cup pesto (homemade or store-bought)
- 1 tbsp olive oil
- 1 tbsp pine nuts (optional)

Serving Size: 1 serving
Nutritional Value: 180 calories, 5g protein, 14g fat, 12g carbs, 3g fiber

Prep Time: 5 minutes
Cook Time: 5 minutes

Instructions:

1. For three to four minutes, sauté zucchini noodles in olive oil.
2. Toss with pesto and top with pine nuts.

Lentil Soup

Ingredients:

- 1 cup lentils
- 1 carrot, diced
- 1 onion, chopped
- 2 garlic cloves, minced
- 4 cups vegetable broth
- 1/2 tsp cumin

Serving Size: 1 serving
Nutritional Value: 250 calories, 15g protein, 4g fat, 45g carbs, 15g fiber

Prep Time: 10 minutes
Cook Time: 30 minutes

Instructions:

1. Sauté onion, garlic, and carrot in a pot for 5 minutes.
2. Add lentils, broth, and cumin, simmer for 30 minutes.

Sweet Potato and Black Bean Tacos

Ingredients:

- 1 small sweet potato, diced
- 1/2 cup black beans, cooked
- 1 whole-wheat tortilla
- 1 tbsp avocado, mashed
- 1 tbsp salsa

Serving Size: 1 serving (2 tacos)
Nutritional Value: 220 calories, 8g protein, 7g fat, 35g carbs, 8g fiber

Prep Time: 10 minutes
Cook Time: 20 minutes

Instructions:

1. Roast sweet potato at 400°F (200°C) for 20 minutes.
2. Warm tortilla, add roasted sweet potato, black beans, mashed avocado, and salsa.

Grilled Veggie Wrap

Ingredients:

- 1 whole-wheat tortilla
- 1/2 cup grilled vegetables (zucchini, bell pepper, mushrooms)
- 1 tbsp hummus

Serving Size: 1 serving
Nutritional Value: 180 calories, 5g protein, 8g fat, 26g carbs, 5g fiber

Prep Time: 5 minutes
Cook Time: 10 minutes

Instructions:

1. Grill vegetables for 5-10 minutes.
2. Spread hummus on tortilla, top with grilled veggies, and wrap.

Cauliflower Rice Stir-Fry

Ingredients:

- 1 cup cauliflower rice
- 1/2 cup mixed vegetables (peas, carrots, bell pepper)
- 1 tbsp soy sauce (low-sodium)
- 1 tsp sesame oil

Serving Size: 1 serving
Nutritional Value: 150 calories, 5g protein, 7g fat, 18g carbs, 6g fiber

Prep Time: 5 minutes
Cook Time: 10 minutes

Instructions:

1. Sauté vegetables in sesame oil for 5 minutes.
2. Add cauliflower rice and soy sauce, cook for another 5 minutes.

Eggplant Parmesan

Ingredients:

- 1 eggplant, sliced
- 1/4 cup breadcrumbs (whole wheat)
- 1/4 cup marinara sauce
- 2 tbsp parmesan cheese

Serving Size: 1 serving
Nutritional Value: 220 calories, 6g protein, 12g fat, 25g carbs, 7g fiber

Prep Time: 10 minutes
Cook Time: 25 minutes

Instructions:

1. Preheat oven to 375°F (190°C).
2. Coat eggplant slices in breadcrumbs, bake for 20 minutes.
3. Top with marinara sauce and parmesan, bake for an additional 5 minutes.

Chickpea Salad

Ingredients:

- 1 cup chickpeas, cooked
- 1/2 cucumber, diced
- 1/4 red onion, diced
- 1 tbsp olive oil
- 1 tbsp lemon juice

Serving Size: 1 serving
Nutritional Value: 220 calories, 10g protein, 8g fat, 28g carbs, 7g fiber

Prep Time: 5 minutes
Cook Time: 0 minutes

Instructions:

1. Mix chickpeas, cucumber, and onion in a bowl.
2. Sprinkle in the lemon juice and olive oil, and mix well.

Vegetable Frittata

Ingredients:

- 2 eggs
- 1/2 cup spinach, chopped
- 1/4 cup bell pepper, diced
- 1/4 cup onion, diced
- 1 tbsp olive oil

Serving Size: 1 serving
Nutritional Value: 220 calories, 14g protein, 14g fat, 10g carbs, 3g fiber

Prep Time: 5 minutes
Cook Time: 10 minutes

Instructions:

1. Sauté onion and bell pepper in olive oil for 3 minutes.
2. Add spinach and beaten eggs, cook until set.

Roasted Brussels Sprouts with Balsamic Vinegar

Ingredients:

- 1 cup Brussels sprouts, halved
- 1 tbsp olive oil
- 1 tbsp balsamic vinegar
- 1/4 tsp black pepper

Serving Size: 1 serving
Nutritional Value: 150 calories, 6g protein, 8g fat, 18g carbs, 7g fiber

Prep Time: 5 minutes
Cook Time: 20 minutes

Instructions:

1. Preheat oven to 400°F (200°C).
2. Toss Brussels sprouts in olive oil, pepper, and balsamic vinegar.
3. Roast for 20 minutes.

Avocado and Tomato Salad

Ingredients:

- 1 avocado, diced
- 1 tomato, diced
- 1 tbsp olive oil
- 1 tbsp lime juice

Serving Size: 1 serving
Nutritional Value: 220 calories, 3g protein, 20g fat, 12g carbs, 9g fiber

Prep Time: 5 minutes
Cook Time: 0 minutes

Instructions:

1. Combine avocado, tomato, olive oil, and lime juice in a bowl.
2. Toss and serve.

Sweet Potato and Kale Salad

Ingredients:

- 1 medium sweet potato, roasted
- 2 cups kale, chopped
- 1 tbsp olive oil
- 1 tbsp apple cider vinegar

Serving Size: 1 serving
Nutritional Value: 230 calories, 4g protein, 10g fat, 34g carbs, 8g fiber

Prep Time: 10 minutes
Cook Time: 20 minutes

Instructions:

1. Roast sweet potato at 400°F (200°C) for 20 minutes.
2. Toss roasted sweet potato with kale, olive oil, and apple cider vinegar.

Butternut Squash Soup

Ingredients:

- 2 cups butternut squash, cubed
- 1 onion, chopped
- 2 garlic cloves, minced
- 3 cups vegetable broth
- 1/2 tsp cinnamon

Serving Size: 1 serving
Nutritional Value: 180 calories, 4g protein, 6g fat, 32g carbs, 6g fiber

Prep Time: 10 minutes
Cook Time: 30 minutes

Instructions:

1. Sauté onion and garlic for 3 minutes.
2. Add squash and vegetable broth, simmer for 30 minutes.
3. Blend until smooth, sprinkle with cinnamon.

Tofu Scramble

Ingredients:

- 1/2 block firm tofu, crumbled
- 1/4 cup bell pepper, diced
- 1/4 cup spinach, chopped
- 1 tbsp olive oil

Serving Size: 1 serving
Nutritional Value: 200 calories, 16g protein, 14g fat, 8g carbs, 3g fiber

Prep Time: 5 minutes
Cook Time: 5 minutes

Instructions:

1. Sauté bell pepper in olive oil for 2 minutes.
2. Add tofu and spinach, cook until warm.

Fruits and Smoothies Recipes

Mango and Spinach Smoothie

Ingredients:

- 1/2 mango, chopped
- 1 cup spinach, fresh
- 1/2 cup almond milk
- 1/2 banana

Serving Size: 1 serving
Nutritional Value: 180 calories, 3g protein, 4g fat, 40g carbs, 5g fiber

Prep Time: 5 minutes
Cook Time: 0 minutes

Instructions:

1. Blend all ingredients until smooth.
2. Serve chilled.

Berry Blast Smoothie

Ingredients:

- 1/2 cup mixed berries (strawberries, blueberries, raspberries)
- 1/2 banana
- 1/2 cup Greek yogurt
- 1/2 cup unsweetened almond milk

Serving Size: 1 serving
Nutritional Value: 150 calories, 8g protein, 2g fat, 25g carbs, 6g fiber

Prep Time: 5 minutes
Cook Time: 0 minutes

Instructions:

1. Combine all ingredients in a blender.

2. Blend until smooth and creamy.

Tropical Avocado Smoothie

Ingredients:

- 1/2 avocado
- 1/2 cup pineapple, chopped
- 1/2 banana
- 1/2 cup coconut water

Serving Size: 1 serving
Nutritional Value: 220 calories, 3g protein, 14g fat, 30g carbs, 8g fiber

Prep Time: 5 minutes
Cook Time: 0 minutes

Instructions:

1. Blend all ingredients until smooth.

2. Serve immediately.

Green Apple and Kale Smoothie

Ingredients:

- 1 green apple, chopped
- 1 cup kale, chopped
- 1/2 banana
- 1/2 cup unsweetened almond milk

Serving Size: 1 serving

Nutritional Value: 180 calories, 3g protein, 2g fat, 40g carbs, 7g fiber

Prep Time: 5 minutes
Cook Time: 0 minutes

Instructions:

1. Blend apple, kale, banana, and almond milk until smooth.
2. Serve chilled.

Watermelon Mint Smoothie

Ingredients:

- 1 cup watermelon, cubed
- 1/4 cup fresh mint leaves
- 1/2 cup unsweetened coconut water
- 1/2 lime, juiced

Serving Size: 1 serving

Nutritional Value: 100 calories, 2g protein, 0g fat, 25g carbs, 3g fiber

Prep Time: 5 minutes
Cook Time: 0 minutes

Instructions:

1. Blend all ingredients until smooth.
2. Serve over ice.

Peach and Banana Smoothie

Ingredients:

- 1/2 peach, chopped
- 1/2 banana
- 1/2 cup Greek yogurt
- 1/2 cup almond milk

Serving Size: 1 serving
Nutritional Value: 170 calories, 7g protein, 2g fat, 33g carbs, 4g fiber

Prep Time: 5 minutes
Cook Time: 0 minutes

Instructions:

1. Blend all ingredients until creamy.
2. Serve immediately.

Pineapple Coconut Smoothie

Ingredients:

- 1/2 cup pineapple, chopped
- 1/2 cup unsweetened coconut milk
- 1 tbsp shredded coconut
- 1/2 banana

Serving Size: 1 serving
Nutritional Value: 160 calories, 2g protein, 8g fat, 30g carbs, 5g fiber

Prep Time: 5 minutes
Cook Time: 0 minutes

Instructions:

1. Blend pineapple, coconut milk, shredded coconut, and banana until smooth.

2. Serve chilled.

Strawberry Banana Smoothie

Ingredients:

- 1/2 cup strawberries

- 1/2 banana

- 1/2 cup Greek yogurt

- 1/2 cup almond milk

Serving Size: 1 serving
Nutritional Value: 150 calories, 8g protein, 3g fat, 30g carbs, 5g fiber

Prep Time: 5 minutes
Cook Time: 0 minutes

Instructions:

1. Blend all ingredients until smooth.

2. Serve immediately.

Blueberry and Oat Smoothie

Ingredients:

- 1/2 cup blueberries
- 1/4 cup rolled oats
- 1/2 banana
- 1/2 cup almond milk

Serving Size: 1 serving
Nutritional Value: 190 calories, 5g protein, 4g fat, 38g carbs, 6g fiber

Prep Time: 5 minutes
Cook Time: 0 minutes

Instructions:

1. Blend blueberries, oats, banana, and almond milk until smooth.
2. Serve chilled.

Mixed Berry Chia Smoothie

Ingredients:

- 1/2 cup mixed berries
- 1 tbsp chia seeds
- 1/2 cup Greek yogurt
- 1/2 cup almond milk

Serving Size: 1 serving
Nutritional Value: 170 calories, 8g protein, 5g fat, 24g carbs, 7g fiber

Prep Time: 5 minutes
Cook Time: 0 minutes

Instructions:

1. Blend all ingredients until smooth.
2. Serve immediately.

Kiwi and Pineapple Smoothie

Ingredients:

- 2 kiwis, peeled
- 1/2 cup pineapple, chopped
- 1/2 cup coconut water

Serving Size: 1 serving
Nutritional Value: 140 calories, 2g protein, 0g fat, 35g carbs, 6g fiber

Prep Time: 5 minutes
Cook Time: 0 minutes

Instructions:

1. Blend kiwis, pineapple, and coconut water until smooth.
2. Serve chilled.

Apple Cinnamon Smoothie

Ingredients:

- 1/2 apple, chopped
- 1/2 banana
- 1/2 tsp cinnamon
- 1/2 cup almond milk

Serving Size: 1 serving
Nutritional Value: 170 calories, 3g protein, 2g fat, 35g carbs, 5g fiber

Prep Time: 5 minutes
Cook Time: 0 minutes

Instructions:

1. Blend apple, banana, cinnamon, and almond milk until smooth.
2. Serve immediately.

Papaya Coconut Smoothie

Ingredients:

- 1/2 papaya, chopped
- 1/2 cup unsweetened coconut milk
- 1/2 banana

Serving Size: 1 serving
Nutritional Value: 180 calories, 2g protein, 8g fat, 35g carbs, 7g fiber

Prep Time: 5 minutes
Cook Time: 0 minutes

Instructions:

1. Blend papaya, coconut milk, and banana until smooth.
2. Serve chilled.

Orange and Carrot Smoothie

Ingredients:

- 1 orange, peeled
- 1/2 carrot, chopped
- 1/2 banana
- 1/2 cup almond milk

Serving Size: 1 serving
Nutritional Value: 160 calories, 2g protein, 2g fat, 35g carbs, 6g fiber

Prep Time: 5 minutes
Cook Time: 0 minutes

Instructions:

1. Blend orange, carrot, banana, and almond milk until smooth.
2. Serve immediately.

Cucumber Mint Smoothie

Ingredients:

- 1/2 cucumber, chopped
- 1/4 cup fresh mint leaves
- 1/2 cup coconut water
- 1/2 lime, juiced

Serving Size: 1 serving
Nutritional Value: 50 calories, 1g protein, 0g fat, 12g carbs, 3g fiber

Prep Time: 5 minutes
Cook Time: 0 minutes

Instructions:

1. Blend cucumber, mint, coconut water, and lime juice until smooth.
2. Serve chilled.

Exercises and Tips

1. Walking

Tip: Walking is one of the simplest and most effective exercises. It is simple, portable, and doesn't require any specialized equipment.

- **Duration:** Start with 20-30 minutes a day, gradually increasing to 60 minutes.
- **Benefit:** Helps lower blood pressure, improve cardiovascular health, and maintain a healthy weight.

2. Strength Training

Tip: Incorporating strength training 2-3 times a week can increase muscle mass and boost metabolism.

- **Exercises:** Squats, lunges, push-ups, and dumbbell exercises.
- **Benefit:** Enhances bone density, increases metabolism, and supports weight loss.

3. Cycling

Tip: Cycling is a low-impact exercise that improves heart health and strengthens leg muscles.

- **Duration:** Aim for 30-60 minutes of moderate-intensity cycling, 3-4 times a week.
- **Benefit:** Burns calories, improves cardiovascular fitness, and boosts leg strength.

4. Swimming

Tip: Swimming is a full-body workout that is easy on the joints.

- **Duration:** Swim for 30 minutes, 3-4 times a week.
- **Benefit:** Builds strength, improves cardiovascular health, and enhances flexibility.

5. Yoga

Tip: Yoga can help with stress reduction, flexibility, and balance.

- **Duration:** Start with 20-30 minutes of yoga sessions, 2-3 times a week.
- **Benefit:** Lowers stress, improves flexibility, and enhances mindfulness.

6. Stretching

Tip: Incorporating daily stretching can improve flexibility and reduce muscle tension.

- **Duration:** Spend 5-10 minutes each day stretching your major muscle groups.
- **Benefit:** Increases flexibility, reduces the risk of injury, and helps with muscle recovery.

7. High-Intensity Interval Training (HIIT)

Tip: HIIT combines short bursts of intense exercise with rest periods, making it an efficient fat-burning workout.

- **Sessions last 20 to 30 minutes each, two to three times a week.**
- **Benefit:** Burns fat quickly, improves cardiovascular health, and boosts metabolism.

8. Pilates

Tip: Pilates focuses on strengthening core muscles, improving posture, and increasing flexibility.

- **Sessions last 20 to 30 minutes each, two to three times a week.**
- **Benefit:** Strengthens the core, improves posture, and enhances flexibility.

9. Climbing Stairs

Tip: If you don't have access to a gym, simply climbing stairs at home or at work can be an excellent workout.

- **Duration:** Climb for 10-15 minutes at a time, 3-4 times a week.

- **Benefit:** Strengthens leg muscles, boosts heart rate, and burns calories.

10. Tai Chi

Tip: Tai Chi is a slow, controlled movement practice that helps with balance and relaxation.

- **Duration:** Practice for 20-30 minutes, 2-3 times a week.
- **Benefit:** Improves balance, reduces stress, and increases flexibility.

11. Dancing

Tip: Dancing is a fun way to get your heart pumping and burn calories.

- **Duration:** Aim for 30 minutes of dancing 2-3 times a week.
- **Benefit:** Improves cardiovascular health, boosts mood, and burns calories.

12. Running or Jogging

Tip: Running is an excellent cardio exercise that helps with weight management and heart health.

- **Duration:** Start with 20-30 minutes of running or jogging, gradually increasing to 45 minutes.
- **Benefit:** Burns fat, improves heart health, and increases stamina.

Exercise Tips:

- **Consistency is Key:** Regular exercise is more effective than sporadic intense sessions.
- **Warm-Up and Cool-Down:** Always warm up before exercises and cool down afterward to prevent injury.
- **Start Slow:** If you're new to exercise, start slowly and gradually increase intensity to avoid overexertion.

- **Mix It Up:** Variety keeps things interesting and works different muscle groups.

- **Stay Hydrated:** Drink plenty of water before, during, and after exercise to stay hydrated.

- **Rest and Recover:** Allow your body time to rest between workouts, especially after strength training or high-intensity exercises.

- **Focus on Form:** Proper technique helps prevent injury and maximizes the effectiveness of your workout.

BONUS

90 Days Healthy Meal Plan

Day	Breakfast	Lunch	Dinner
1	Oatmeal with Berries	Grilled Chicken Salad	Baked Salmon with Quinoa
2	Avocado Toast with Eggs	Turkey & Avocado Wrap	Lentil Soup with Veggies
3	Greek Yogurt with Honey & Almonds	Spinach & Feta Salad with Chicken	Grilled Shrimp with Asparagus
4	Whole Wheat Pancakes with Berries	Tuna Salad on Whole Wheat Bread	Baked Chicken with Sweet Potato
5	Scrambled Eggs with Spinach & Tomatoes	Quinoa & Black Bean Salad	Grilled Cod with Veggie Stir-Fry
6	Chia Seed Pudding with Fruit	Chickpea & Cucumber Salad	Stir-fried Tofu with Vegetables
7	Smoothie with Spinach & Banana	Roasted Veggie Salad with Hummus	Grilled Chicken with Steamed Broccoli
8	Whole Wheat Toast with Almond Butter	Turkey Sandwich with Spinach & Avocado	Salmon with Roasted Brussels Sprouts
9	Greek Yogurt with Strawberries	Grilled Veggie Wrap	Zucchini Noodles with Marinara

Day	Breakfast	Lunch	Dinner
10	Scrambled Eggs with Bell Peppers	Quinoa Salad with Roasted Veggies	Chicken Stir-Fry with Veggies
11	Oatmeal with Walnuts & Cinnamon	Grilled Chicken Caesar Salad	Baked Cod with Roasted Potatoes
12	Whole Wheat Bagel with Cream Cheese	Chicken & Avocado Salad	Lentil Stew with Veggies
13	Smoothie with Mango & Spinach	Grilled Salmon Salad	Roasted Chicken with Carrots
14	Veggie Omelet with Whole Wheat Toast	Quinoa with Roasted Sweet Potatoes	Grilled Shrimp with Brown Rice
15	Avocado Toast with Tomato & Eggs	Mediterranean Salad with Chicken	Grilled Pork Chops with Roasted Veggies
16	Whole Wheat Pancakes with Banana	Lentil & Veggie Salad	Stir-fried Tofu with Broccoli
17	Chia Seed Pudding with Blueberries	Turkey Wrap with Veggies	Grilled Salmon with Spinach
18	Oatmeal with Apples & Cinnamon	Quinoa Salad with Spinach	Chicken & Veggie Skewers
19	Smoothie with Berries & Almond Milk	Grilled Veggie Salad with Hummus	Salmon with Cauliflower Rice

Day	Breakfast	Lunch	Dinner
20	Scrambled Eggs with Spinach & Mushrooms	Chickpea & Tomato Salad	Baked Chicken with Sweet Potato
21	Greek Yogurt with Walnuts & Honey	Chicken Caesar Salad	Grilled Shrimp with Veggies
22	Whole Wheat Toast with Peanut Butter	Grilled Veggie Wrap	Zucchini Noodles with Garlic & Olive Oil
23	Scrambled Eggs with Avocado	Turkey & Spinach Salad	Lentil Soup with Veggies
24	Whole Wheat Bagel with Cream Cheese	Tuna Salad with Cucumber & Tomato	Grilled Chicken with Quinoa
25	Oatmeal with Blueberries	Grilled Chicken Salad	Baked Salmon with Roasted Veggies
26	Smoothie with Banana & Almond Butter	Quinoa Salad with Veggies	Stir-fried Tofu with Rice
27	Veggie Omelet with Tomatoes & Bell Peppers	Grilled Veggie Wrap	Chicken Stir-Fry with Veggies
28	Greek Yogurt with Strawberries	Turkey & Avocado Sandwich	Salmon with Roasted Sweet Potatoes
29	Whole Wheat Pancakes with Apples	Grilled Chicken Salad with Veggies	Lentil Stew with Veggies

Day	Breakfast	Lunch	Dinner
30	Chia Seed Pudding with Almonds	Grilled Salmon with Veggies	Roasted Pork with Roasted Vegetables

Day	Breakfast	Lunch	Dinner
31	Oatmeal with Berries	Chicken Salad with Tomatoes	Grilled Salmon with Asparagus
32	Smoothie with Spinach & Apple	Grilled Veggie Wrap	Chicken & Veggie Stir-Fry
33	Scrambled Eggs with Spinach	Tuna Salad with Mixed Greens	Baked Chicken with Sweet Potato
34	Whole Wheat Pancakes with Bananas	Mediterranean Chicken Salad	Grilled Shrimp with Brown Rice
35	Veggie Omelet with Whole Wheat Toast	Grilled Veggie & Hummus Wrap	Chicken Stir-Fry with Veggies
36	Chia Seed Pudding with Fruit	Quinoa Salad with Chicken	Grilled Salmon with Broccoli
37	Greek Yogurt with Berries	Turkey & Spinach Salad	Stir-fried Tofu with Veggies

Day	Breakfast	Lunch	Dinner
38	Whole Wheat Toast with Avocado	Grilled Veggie Salad with Chicken	Grilled Pork Chops with Veggies
39	Smoothie with Mango & Spinach	Lentil & Veggie Soup	Roasted Chicken with Carrots
40	Oatmeal with Walnuts & Cinnamon	Tuna Salad on Whole Wheat Bread	Grilled Salmon with Roasted Veggies
41	Scrambled Eggs with Tomatoes	Chicken Caesar Salad	Baked Chicken with Sweet Potatoes
42	Greek Yogurt with Almonds	Quinoa Salad with Veggies	Grilled Shrimp with Cauliflower Rice
43	Whole Wheat Bagel with Cream Cheese	Grilled Chicken Wrap	Veggie Stir-Fry with Tofu
44	Chia Seed Pudding with Strawberries	Grilled Salmon Salad	Roasted Chicken with Sweet Potatoes
45	Smoothie with Berries & Almond Milk	Quinoa Salad with Veggies	Stir-fried Tofu with Vegetables
46	Veggie Omelet with Whole Wheat Toast	Roasted Veggie Salad with Chickpeas	Grilled Pork Chops with Roasted Veggies
47	Oatmeal with Blueberries	Turkey & Avocado Wrap	Chicken & Veggie Skewers

Day	Breakfast	Lunch	Dinner
48	Greek Yogurt with Honey & Almonds	Grilled Chicken with Veggies	Grilled Shrimp with Veggie Stir-Fry
49	Scrambled Eggs with Bell Peppers	Chicken Caesar Salad	Baked Salmon with Sweet Potatoes
50	Whole Wheat Toast with Peanut Butter	Lentil Soup with Veggies	Grilled Chicken with Roasted Veggies
51	Smoothie with Spinach & Banana	Grilled Veggie Salad	Stir-fried Tofu with Brown Rice
52	Veggie Omelet with Whole Wheat Toast	Grilled Chicken Wrap	Grilled Salmon with Cauliflower Rice
53	Oatmeal with Walnuts & Cinnamon	Mediterranean Quinoa Salad	Baked Chicken with Roasted Potatoes
54	Scrambled Eggs with Spinach & Mushrooms	Quinoa Salad with Veggies	Stir-fried Chicken with Veggies
55	Whole Wheat Bagel with Cream Cheese	Grilled Veggie Wrap	Grilled Shrimp with Roasted Veggies
56	Smoothie with Berries & Almond Milk	Grilled Chicken Salad	Stir-fried Tofu with Brown Rice
57	Chia Seed Pudding with Blueberries	Lentil Soup with Veggies	Grilled Pork Chops with Sweet Potatoes

Day	Breakfast	Lunch	Dinner
58	Greek Yogurt with Honey & Walnuts	Quinoa Salad with Veggies	Grilled Shrimp with Steamed Broccoli
59	Oatmeal with Strawberries	Grilled Veggie Salad with Avocado	Chicken & Veggie Stir-Fry
60	Whole Wheat Pancakes with Apples	Grilled Chicken Caesar Salad	Roasted Salmon with Veggies

Day	Breakfast	Lunch	Dinner
61	Greek Yogurt with Berries	Roasted Veggie & Hummus Wrap	Baked Salmon with Quinoa
62	Scrambled Eggs with Spinach	Chicken Caesar Salad	Grilled Shrimp with Cauliflower Rice
63	Whole Wheat Toast with Peanut Butter	Lentil Soup with Veggies	Stir-fried Chicken with Veggies
64	Oatmeal with Banana & Cinnamon	Grilled Chicken Salad	Grilled Pork Chops with Roasted Veggies
65	Veggie Omelet with Whole Wheat Toast	Tuna Salad with Mixed Greens	Baked Chicken with Sweet Potato

Day	Breakfast	Lunch	Dinner
66	Chia Seed Pudding with Strawberries	Grilled Veggie Wrap	Grilled Salmon with Broccoli
67	Smoothie with Mango & Almond Milk	Grilled Shrimp Salad	Chicken Stir-Fry with Veggies
68	Scrambled Eggs with Tomatoes	Mediterranean Quinoa Salad	Roasted Pork Chops with Sweet Potatoes
69	Greek Yogurt with Strawberries	Grilled Veggie Salad	Grilled Shrimp with Veggies
70	Oatmeal with Walnuts & Cinnamon	Grilled Chicken with Veggies	Stir-fried Tofu with Veggies
71	Whole Wheat Pancakes with Bananas	Tuna Salad with Mixed Greens	Baked Chicken with Sweet Potatoes
72	Scrambled Eggs with Spinach	Lentil Soup with Veggies	Grilled Salmon with Asparagus
73	Chia Seed Pudding with Blueberries	Grilled Chicken Wrap	Stir-fried Tofu with Vegetables
74	Greek Yogurt with Almonds	Grilled Veggie Salad	Roasted Chicken with Carrots
75	Whole Wheat Toast with Avocado	Quinoa Salad with Veggies	Grilled Shrimp with Brown Rice

Day	Breakfast	Lunch	Dinner
76	Oatmeal with Strawberries	Chicken Caesar Salad	Grilled Salmon with Roasted Sweet Potatoes
77	Smoothie with Spinach & Banana	Mediterranean Quinoa Salad	Baked Chicken with Veggies
78	Whole Wheat Bagel with Cream Cheese	Lentil Soup with Veggies	Stir-fried Chicken with Veggies
79	Greek Yogurt with Honey & Almonds	Roasted Veggie Salad with Chickpeas	Grilled Salmon with Quinoa
80	Smoothie with Mango & Almond Butter	Quinoa Salad with Veggies	Grilled Shrimp with Veggies
81	Oatmeal with Walnuts & Cinnamon	Grilled Chicken Salad	Baked Salmon with Roasted Veggies
82	Scrambled Eggs with Avocado	Tuna Salad with Mixed Greens	Grilled Chicken with Quinoa
83	Whole Wheat Pancakes with Apples	Mediterranean Chicken Salad	Stir-fried Tofu with Vegetables
84	Chia Seed Pudding with Fruit	Grilled Veggie Wrap	Grilled Shrimp with Roasted Sweet Potatoes
85	Oatmeal with Banana & Cinnamon	Lentil Soup with Veggies	Grilled Pork Chops with Roasted Potatoes

Day	Breakfast	Lunch	Dinner
86	Veggie Omelet with Spinach & Tomatoes	Grilled Chicken Salad	Stir-fried Tofu with Brown Rice
87	Greek Yogurt with Honey & Almonds	Grilled Veggie Salad	Grilled Shrimp with Veggies
88	Whole Wheat Bagel with Cream Cheese	Quinoa Salad with Roasted Veggies	Baked Salmon with Sweet Potato
89	Oatmeal with Strawberries	Grilled Veggie Wrap	Stir-fried Chicken with Veggies
90	Chia Seed Pudding with Berries	Roasted Veggie & Hummus Wrap	Grilled Pork Chops with Veggies

Printed in Great Britain
by Amazon